The Concise Book
of Trigger Points

The Concise Book of Trigger Points

Simeon Niel-Asher

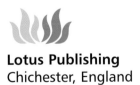

Lotus Publishing
Chichester, England

North Atlantic Books
Berkeley, California

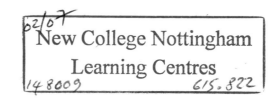

First published in 2005 and reprinted with corrections in 2006 by
Lotus Publishing
3 Chapel Street, Chichester, PO19 1BU and
North Atlantic Books
P O Box 12327
Berkeley, California 94712

Anatomical Drawings Amanda Williams
Line Drawings Chris Fulcher
Text and Cover Design Chris Fulcher
Printed and Bound in the UK by Scotprint

The Concise Book of Trigger Points is sponsored by the Society for the Study of Native Arts and Sciences, a nonprofit educational corporation whose goals are to develop an educational and crosscultural perspective linking various scientific, social, and artistic fields; to nurture a holistic view of arts, sciences, humanities, and healing; and to publish and distribute literature on the relationship of mind, body, and nature.

Dedication
With thanks to my wife, family and wonderful patients for their ongoing love, friendship and support.

British Library Cataloguing in Publication Data
A CIP record for this book is available from the British Library
ISBN 0 9543188 5 4 (Lotus Publishing)
ISBN 1 55643 536 3 (North Atlantic Books)

Library of Congress Cataloging-in-Publication Data

Niel-Asher, Simeon.
   The concise book of trigger points / by Simeon Niel-Asher.
      p. ; cm.
   Includes bibliographical references and index.
   Summary: "A manual for understanding and treating chronic pain associated with trigger points, the tender, painful nodules that form in muscles and connective tissues"--Provided by publisher.
   ISBN 1-55643-536-3 (pbk.)
   1. Myofascial pain syndromes--Treatment--Handbooks, manuals, etc. 2. Chronic disease--Treatment--Handbooks, manuals, etc. I. Title.
   [DNLM: 1. Myofascial Pain Syndromes--therapy--Handbooks. 2. Chronic Disease--therapy--Handbooks. 3. Myofascial Pain Syndromes--physiopathology--Handbooks.   WE 39 N667c 2005]
   RC927.3.N45 2005
   616.7'4--dc22

2005024075

Contents

About this Book

This book is designed in quick reference format to offer useful information about the trigger points relating to the main skeletal muscles, that are central to massage, bodywork, and physical therapy. Each muscle section is colour-coded for ease of reference. Enough detail is included regarding each muscle's origin, insertion, innervation, and action commensurate with the requirements of the student and practitioner. The information about each muscle is presented in a uniform style throughout. An example is given below, with the meaning of headings explained in bold (some muscles will have abbreviated versions of this).

It must be noted that locating a trigger point within a muscle is not an exact science. The typical, and standard practice in all books to date is to include an X to identify the location of a trigger point. However, the concept of X marks the spot may be misleading. Trigger points tend to develop in the muscle belly, in the region of the motor neurone end plate. Where possible, I have indicated the most common location of the central trigger points. It is important to note that these points are not 'fixed'; they are for indication purposes only. In the clinical setting you may well find the trigger point location varies. Varying the direction, amplitude and applicator force will also have an impact on locating the trigger point.

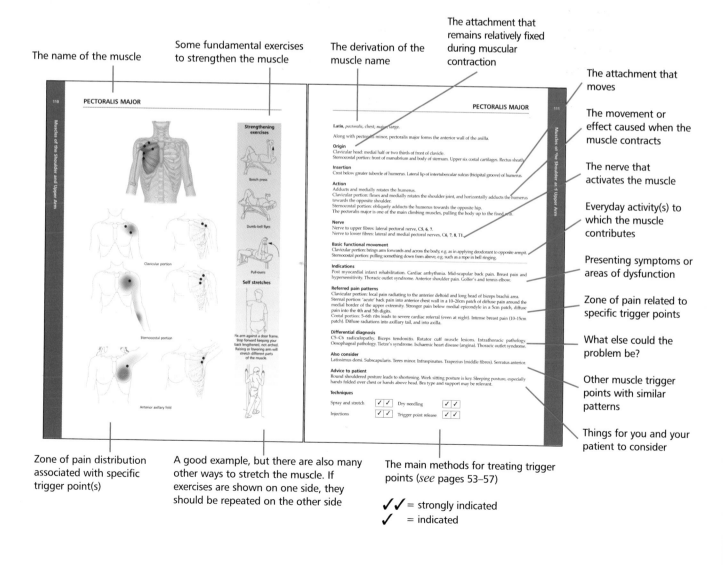

The name of the muscle

Some fundamental exercises to strengthen the muscle

The derivation of the muscle name

The attachment that remains relatively fixed during muscular contraction

The attachment that moves

The movement or effect caused when the muscle contracts

The nerve that activates the muscle

Everyday activity(s) to which the muscle contributes

Presenting symptoms or areas of dysfunction

Zone of pain related to specific trigger points

What else could the problem be?

Other muscle trigger points with similar patterns

Things for you and your patient to consider

Zone of pain distribution associated with specific trigger point(s)

A good example, but there are also many other ways to stretch the muscle. If exercises are shown on one side, they should be repeated on the other side

The main methods for treating trigger points (*see* pages 53–57)

✓✓ = strongly indicated
✓ = indicated

A Note About Peripheral Nerve Supply

The nervous system comprises:

• The central nervous system (i.e. the brain and spinal cord).
• The peripheral nervous system (including the autonomic nervous system, i.e. all neural structures outside the brain and spinal cord).

The peripheral nervous system consists of 12 pairs of cranial nerves and 31 pairs of spinal nerves (with their subsequent branches). The spinal nerves are numbered according to the level of the spinal cord from which they arise (the level is known as the spinal segment).

The relevant peripheral nerve supply is listed with each muscle presented in this book, for those who need to know. However, information about the spinal segment* from which the nerve fibres emanate often differs between the various sources. This is because it is extremely difficult for anatomists to trace the route of an individual nerve fibre through the intertwining maze of other nerve fibres as it passes through its plexus (plexus = a network of nerves: from the Latin word meaning 'braid'). Therefore, such information has been derived mainly from empirical clinical observation, rather than through dissection of the body.

In order to give the most accurate information possible, I have followed the idea of Chris Jarmey, and duplicated the method devised by Florence Peterson Kendall and Elizabeth Kendall McCreary (*see* resources: Muscles Testing and Function). Kendall & McCreary integrated information from six well-known anatomy reference texts; namely, those written by: Cunningham, deJong, Foerster & Bumke, Gray, Haymaker & Woodhall, and Spalteholz. Following the same procedure, and then cross-matching the results with those of Kendall & McCreary, the following system of emphasising the most important nerve roots for each muscle has been adopted in this book.

Let us take the supinator muscle as our example, which is supplied by the deep radial nerve, C5, **6**, (7). The relevant spinal segment is indicated by the letter [C] and the numbers [5, **6**, (7)]. Bold numbers [e.g. **6**] indicate that most (at least five) of the sources agree. Numbers that are not bold [e.g. 5] reflect agreement by three of four sources. Numbers not in bold and in parenthesis [e.g. (7)] reflect agreement by two sources only, or if more than two sources specifically regarded it as a very minimal supply. If a spinal segment was mentioned by only one source, it was disregarded. Hence, bold type indicates the major innervation; not bold indicates the minor innervation; and numbers in parenthesis suggest possible or infrequent innervation.

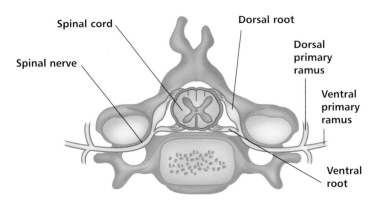

Figure 1: A spinal segment, showing the nerve roots combining to form a spinal nerve, which then divides into ventral and dorsal rami.

*A spinal segment is the part of the spinal cord that gives rise to each pair of spinal nerves (a pair consists of one nerve for the left side and one for the right side of the body). Each spinal nerve contains motor and sensory fibres. Soon after the spinal nerve exits through the foramen (the opening between adjacent vertebrae), it divides into a dorsal primary ramus (directed posteriorly) and a ventral primary ramus (directed laterally or anteriorly). Fibres from the dorsal rami innervate the skin and extensor muscles of the neck and trunk. The ventral rami supply the limbs, plus the sides and front of the trunk.

1

The Moving Body

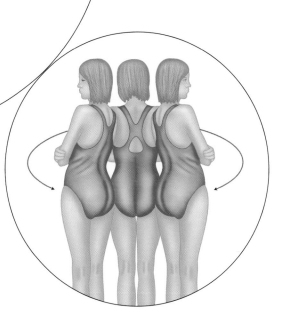

Anatomical Directions

To describe the relative position of body parts and their movements, it is essential to have a universally accepted initial reference position. The standard body position known as the anatomical position serves as this reference. The *anatomical position* is simply the upright standing position with arms hanging by the sides, palms facing forwards (*see* figure 1.1). Most directional terminology used refers to the body *as if* it were in the anatomical position, regardless of its actual position. Note also that the terms 'left' or 'right' refer to the sides of the object or person being viewed, and not those of the reader.

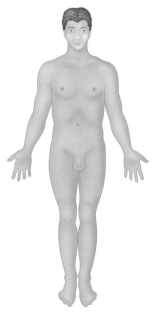

Figure 1.1: **Anterior**
In front of; toward or at the front of the body.

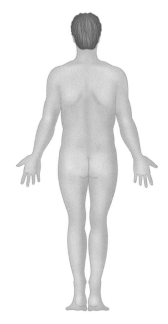

Figure 1.2: **Posterior**
Behind; toward or at the backside of the body.

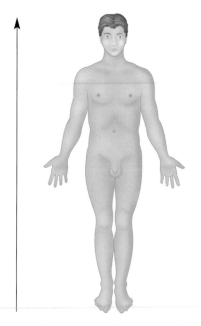

Figure 1.3: **Superior**
Above; toward the head or upper part
of the structure or the body.

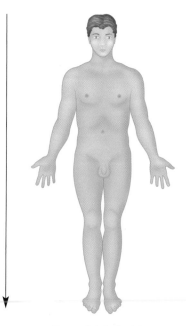

Figure 1.4: **Inferior**
Below; away from the head or toward the
lower part of a structure or the body.

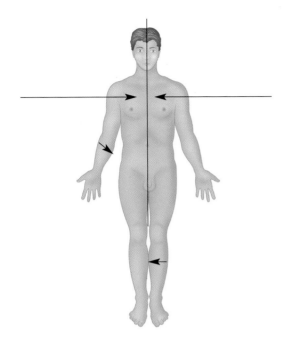

Figure 1.5: **Medial**
(from *medius* in Latin, meaning middle). Toward or at the midline of the body; on the inner side of a limb.

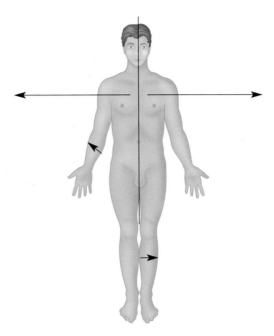

Figure 1.6: **Lateral**
(from *latus* in Latin, meaning side). Away from the midline of the body; on the outer side of the body or a limb.

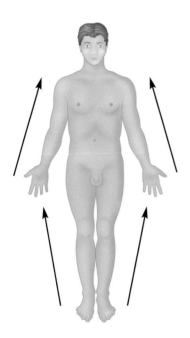

Figure 1.7: **Proximal**
(from *proximus* in Latin, meaning next to). Closer to the centre of the body (the navel), or to the point of attachment of a limb to the body torso.

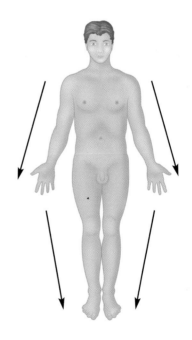

Figure 1.8: **Distal**
(from *distans* in Latin, meaning distant). Farther from the centre of the body, or from the point of attachment of a limb to the torso.

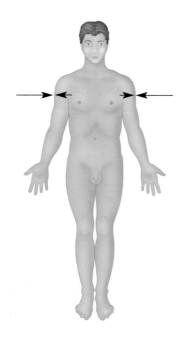

Figure 1.9: **Superficial**
Toward or at the body surface.

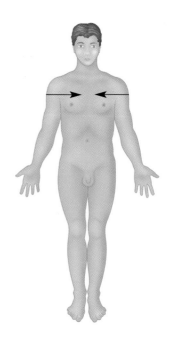

Figure 1.10: **Deep**
Farther away from the body surface; more internal.

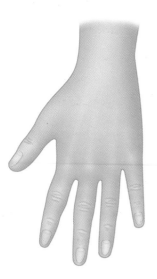

Figure 1.11: **Dorsum**
The posterior surface of something,
e.g. the back of the hand;
the top of the foot.

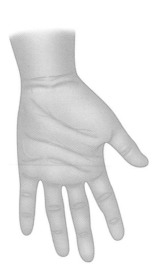

Figure 1.12: **Palmar**
The anterior surface of the hand,
i.e. the palm.

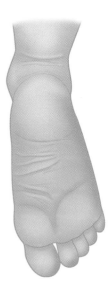

Figure 1.13: **Plantar**
The sole of the foot.

Regional Areas

The two primary divisions of the body are its *axial* part, consisting of the head, neck and trunk, and its *appendicular* parts, consisting of the limbs that are attached to the axis of the body. Figure 1.14 shows the terms used to indicate specific body areas. Terms enclosed within brackets refer to the lay term for the area.

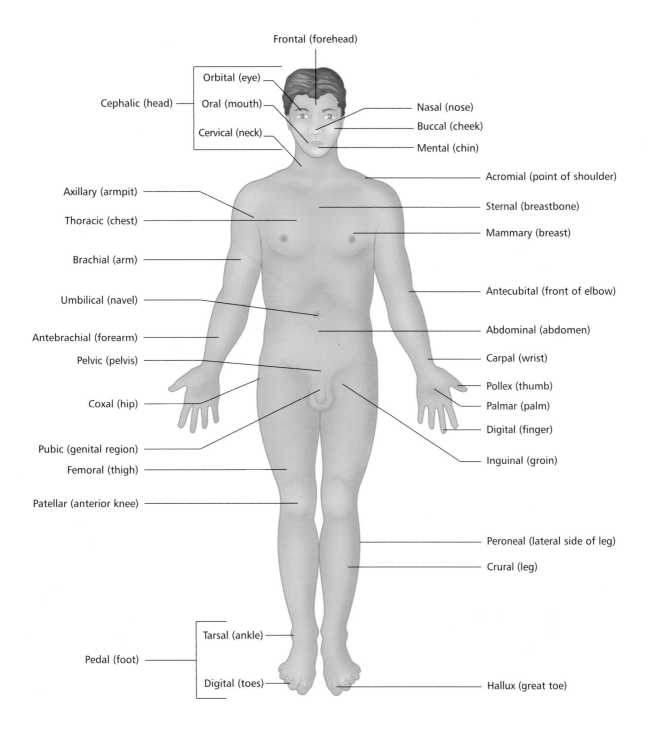

Figure 1.14: Terms used to indicate specific body areas; a) anterior view.

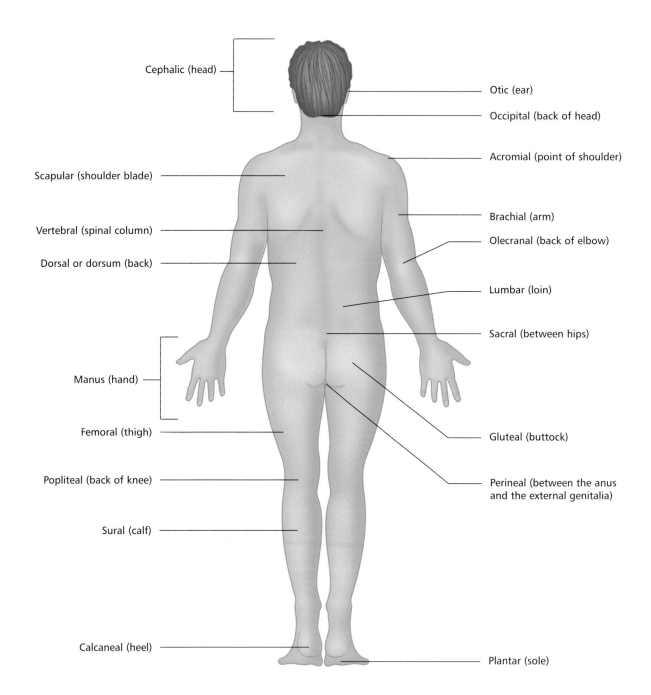

Cephalic (head)

Otic (ear)

Occipital (back of head)

Acromial (point of shoulder)

Scapular (shoulder blade)

Brachial (arm)

Vertebral (spinal column)

Olecranal (back of elbow)

Dorsal or dorsum (back)

Lumbar (loin)

Sacral (between hips)

Manus (hand)

Femoral (thigh)

Gluteal (buttock)

Popliteal (back of knee)

Perineal (between the anus and the external genitalia)

Sural (calf)

Calcaneal (heel)

Plantar (sole)

Figure 1.14: Terms used to indicate specific body areas; b) posterior view.

Planes of the Body

Planes refer to two-dimensional sections through the body, to give a view of the body or body part, as if it has been cut through an imaginary line.

- The sagittal planes cut vertically through the body from anterior to posterior, dividing the body into right and left halves. The illustration shows the mid-sagittal plane.

- The frontal (coronal) planes pass vertically through the body, dividing the body into anterior and posterior sections, and lies at right angles to the sagittal plane.

- The transverse planes are horizontal cross sections, dividing the body into upper (superior) and lower (inferior) sections, and lie at right angles to the other two planes. Figure 1.15 illustrates the most frequently used planes.

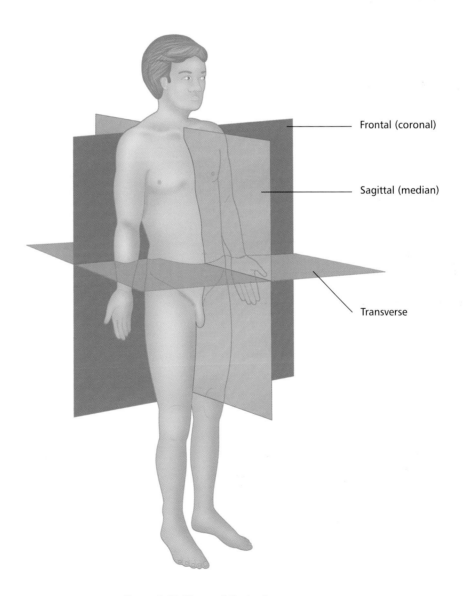

Figure 1.15: Planes of the body.

Anatomical Movements

The direction that body parts move is described in relation to the foetal (fetal) position. Moving into the foetal position results from flexion of all the limbs. Straightening out of the foetal position results from extension of all the limbs.

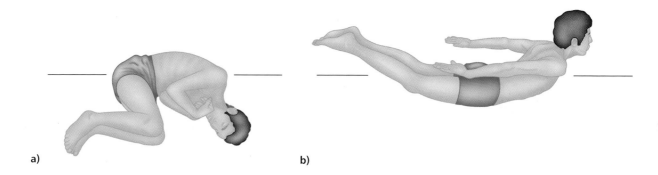

a)

b)

Figure 1.16: a) Flexion into the foetal position; b) extension out of the foetal position.

Main Movements

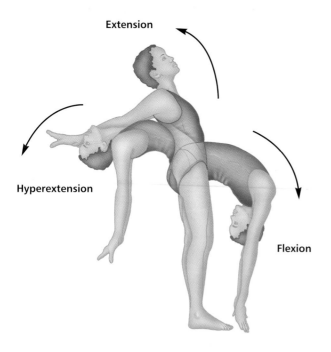

Extension

Hyperextension

Flexion

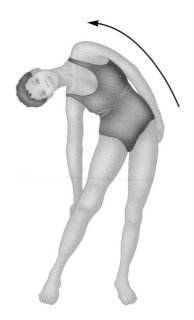

Figure 1.17: **Flexion**: Bending to decrease the angle between bones at a joint. From the anatomical position, flexion is usually forward, except at the knee joint where it is backward. The way to remember this is that flexion is always toward the foetal position. **Extension**: To straighten or bend backward away from the foetal position. **Hyperextension**: To extend the limb beyond its normal range.

Figure 1.18: **Lateral flexion**
To bend the torso or head laterally (sideways) in the frontal (coronal) plane.

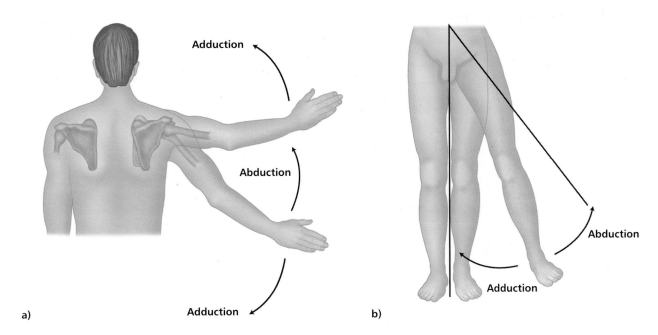

Figure 1.19a and b:
Abduction: Movement of a bone away from the midline of the body, or the midline of a limb.
Adduction: Movement of a bone towards the midline of the body, or the midline of a limb.

NOTE: for abduction of the arm to continue above the height of the shoulder (elevation through abduction), the scapula must rotate on its axis to turn the glenoid cavity upwards (*see* figure 1.27b).

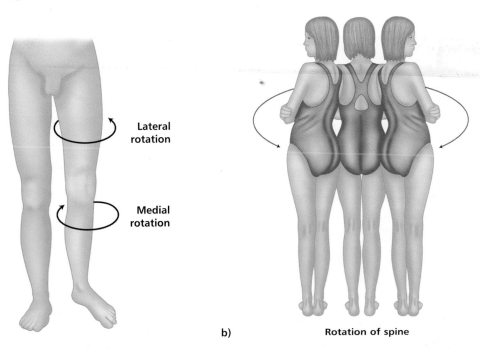

Figure 1.20:
Rotation: Movement of a bone or the trunk around its own longitudinal axis.
Medial rotation: to turn in towards the midline.
Lateral rotation: to turn out, away from the midline.

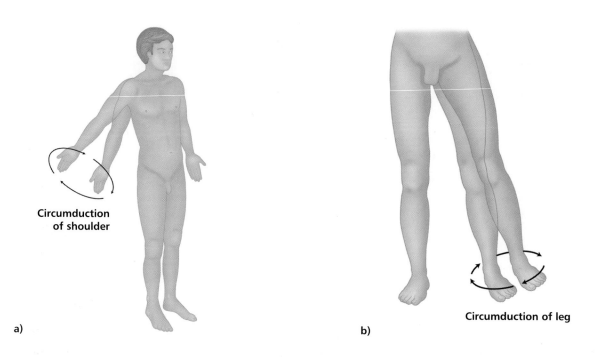

Circumduction of shoulder

a)

Circumduction of leg

b)

Figure 1.21: **Circumduction**
Movement in which the distal end of a bone moves in a circle, while the proximal end remains stable;
the movement combines flexion, abduction, extension, and adduction.

Other Movements

Movements in this section are those that occur only at specific joints or parts of the body; usually involving more than one joint.

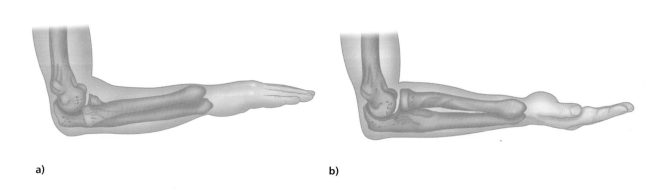

a)

b)

Figure 1.22a: **Pronation**
To turn the palm of the hand down to face the floor
(if standing with elbow bent 90°, or if lying flat on the
floor), or away from the anatomical and foetal positions.

Figure 1.22b: **Supination**
To turn the palm of the hand up to face the ceiling
(if standing with elbow bent 90°, or if lying flat on the
floor), or toward the anatomical and foetal positions.

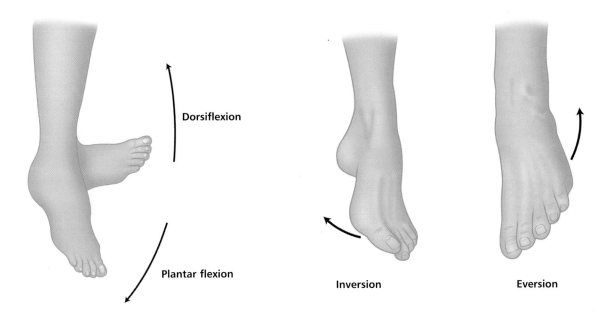

Figure 1.23: **Plantar flexion**: To point the toes down towards the ground. **Dorsiflexion**: To point the toes up towards the sky.

Figure 1.24: **Inversion**: To turn the sole of the foot inward, so that the soles would face towards each other. **Eversion**: To turn the sole of the foot outward, so that the soles would face away from each other.

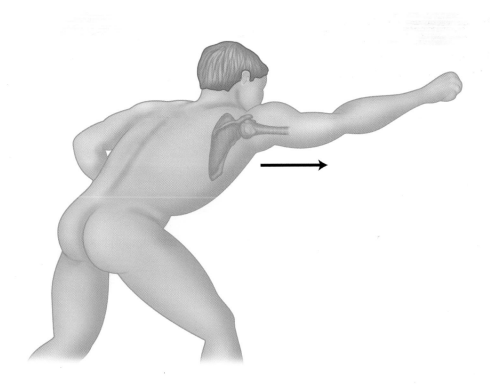

Figure 1.25: **Protraction**
Movement forwards in the transverse plane.
For example, protraction of the shoulder girdle, as in rounding the shoulder.

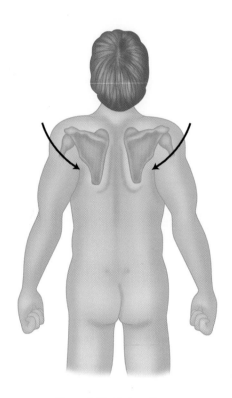

Figure 1.26: **Retraction**
Movement backwards in the transverse plane,
as in bracing the shoulder girdle back, military style.

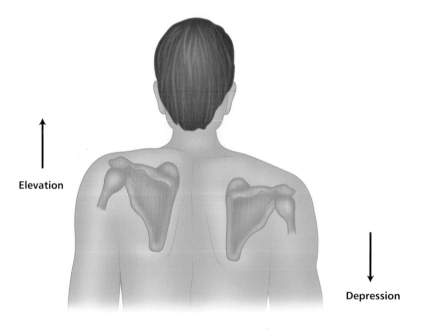

Figure 1.27a:
Elevation: Movement of a part of the body upwards along the frontal plane.
For example, elevating the scapula by shrugging the shoulders.
Depression: Movement of an elevated part of the body downwards to its original position.

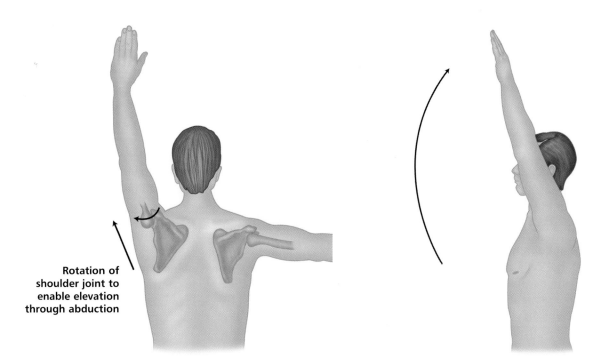

Rotation of
shoulder joint to
enable elevation
through abduction

Figure 1.27b: Abducting the arm at the shoulder joint, then
continuing to raise it above the head in the frontal plane
can be referred to as **elevation through abduction**.

Figure 1.27c: Flexing the arm at the shoulder joint, then
continuing to raise it above the head in the sagittal plane
can be referred to as **elevation through flexion**.

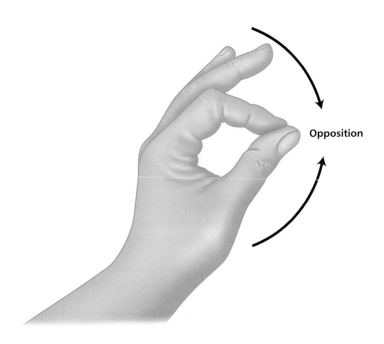

Opposition

Figure 1.28: **Opposition**
A movement specific to the saddle joint of the thumb,
that enables you to touch your thumb to the tips of the fingers of the same hand.

Skeletal Muscle

Red and White Muscle Fibres

There are *three* types of skeletal muscle fibres: red slow-twitch fibres, white fast-twitch fibres, and intermediate fast-twitch fibres.

1. Red Slow-twitch Fibres
These are thin cells that contract slowly. The red colour is due to their content of myoglobin, a substance similar to haemoglobin, which stores oxygen and increases the rate of oxygen diffusion within the muscle fibre. As long as oxygen supply is plentiful, red fibres can contract for sustained periods, and are thus very resistant to fatigue. Successful marathon runners tend to have a high percentage of these red fibres.

2. White Fast-twitch Fibres
These are large cells that contract rapidly. They are pale, due to a lesser content of myoglobin. They fatigue quickly, because they rely on short-lived glycogen reserves in the fibre to contract. However, they are capable of generating much more powerful contractions than red fibres, enabling them to perform rapid, powerful movements for short periods. Successful sprinters have a higher proportion of these white fibres.

3. Intermediate Fast-twitch Fibres
These red or pink fibres are a compromise in size and activity between the red and white fibres.

NOTE: There is always a mixture of these muscle fibres in any given muscle, giving them a range of fatigue resistance and contractile speeds.

Blood Supply

In general, each muscle receives one artery to *bring* nutrients via blood into the muscle, and several veins, to *take away* metabolic waste products surrendered by the muscle into the blood. These blood vessels generally enter through the central part of the muscle, but can also enter towards one end. Thereafter, they branch into a capillary plexus, which spreads throughout the intermuscular septa, to eventually penetrate the endomysium around each muscle fibre. During exercise the capillaries dilate, increasing the amount of blood flow in the muscle by up to 800 times. The muscle tendon, because it is composed of a relatively inactive tissue, has a much less extensive blood supply.

Nerve Supply

The nerve supply to a muscle usually enters at the same place as the blood supply, and branches through the connective tissue septa into the endomysium in a similar way. Each skeletal muscle fibre is supplied by a single nerve ending. This is in contrast to other muscle tissues, which are able to contract without any nerve stimulation.

The nerve entering the muscle usually contains roughly equal proportions of sensory and motor nerve fibres, although some muscles may receive separate sensory branches. As the nerve fibre approaches the muscle fibre, it divides into a number of terminal branches, collectively called a *motor end plate*.

Motor Unit of a Skeletal Muscle

A motor unit consists of a single motor nerve cell and the muscle fibres stimulated by it. The motor units vary in size, ranging from cylinders of muscle 5–7mm in diameter in the upper limb and 7–10mm in diameter in the lower limb. The average number of muscle fibres within a unit is 150 (but this number ranges from less than 10 to several hundred). Where fine gradations of movement are required, as in the muscles of the eyeball or fingers, the number of muscle fibres supplied by a single nerve cell is small. On the other hand, where more gross movements are required, as in the muscles of the lower limb, each nerve cell may supply a motor unit of several hundred fibres.

The muscle fibres in a single motor unit are spread throughout the muscle, rather than being clustered together. This means that stimulation of a single motor unit will cause the entire muscle to exhibit a weak contraction.

Skeletal muscles work on an '*All or Nothing Principle*'. In other words, groups of muscle cells, or fasciculi, can either contract or not contract. Depending on the strength of contraction required, a certain number of muscle cells will contract totally, while others will not contract at all. When a great muscular effort is needed, most of the motor units may be stimulated at the same time. However, under normal conditions, the motor units tend to work in relays, so that during prolonged contractions some are resting while others are contracting.

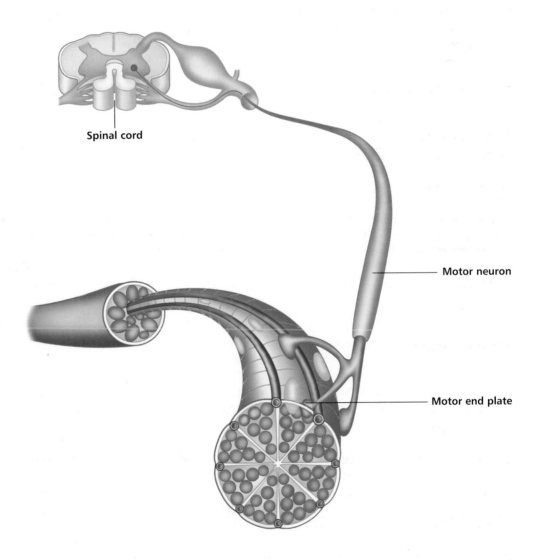

Spinal cord

Motor neuron

Motor end plate

Figure 1.29: A motor unit of a skeletal muscle.

Muscle Shape (Arrangement of Fascicles)

Muscle shape is of direct relevance to trigger points; the shape determining the distribution and quantity. Muscles come in a variety of shapes according to the arrangement of their fascicles. The reason for this variation is to provide optimum mechanical efficiency for a muscle in relation to its position and action. The most common arrangement of fascicles give muscle shapes described as parallel, pennate, convergent and circular. Each of these shapes has further sub-categories.

Parallel

This arrangement has the fascicles running parallel to the long axis of the muscle. If the fascicles extend throughout the length of the muscle, it is known as a *strap muscle*, for example: sartorius (*see* figure 1.30). If the muscle also has an expanded belly and tendons at both ends, it is called a *fusiform* muscle, for example, the biceps brachii of the arm (*see* figure 1.30). A modification of this type of muscle has a fleshy belly at either end, with a tendon in the middle. Such muscles are referred to as *digastric*, e.g. digastricus (*see* figure 1.30).

Pennate

Pennate muscles are so named because their short fasciculi are attached obliquely to the tendon, like the structure of a feather (penna = feather). If the tendon develops on one side of the muscle, it is referred to as *unipennate*, for example, the flexor digitorum longus in the leg (*see* figure 1.30). If the tendon is in the middle and fibres are attached obliquely from both sides, it is known as *bipennate*, of which the rectus femoris is a good example (*see* figure 1.30). If there are numerous tendinous intrusions into the muscle with fibres attaching obliquely from several directions, thus resembling many feathers side by side, the muscle is referred to as *multipennate*; the best example being the middle part of the deltoid muscle (*see* figure 1.30).

Convergent

Muscles that have a broad origin with fascicles converging toward a single tendon, giving the muscle a triangular shape, are called *convergent* muscles. The best example is the pectoralis major (*see* figure 1.30).

Circular

When the fascicles of a muscle are arranged in concentric rings, the muscle is referred to as *circular*. All the sphincter skeletal muscles in the body are of this type; i.e. they surround openings, which they close by contracting. An example includes the orbicularis oculi (*see* figure 1.30).

When a muscle contracts, it can shorten by up to 70% of its original length. Hence, the longer the fibres, the greater the range of movement. On the other hand, the strength of a muscle depends on the total number of muscle fibres it contains, rather than their length. Therefore:

1. Muscles with long parallel fibres produce the greatest range of movement, but are not usually very powerful.

2. Muscles with a pennate pattern, especially if multipennate, pack in the most fibres. Such muscles shorten less than long parallel muscles, but tend to be much more powerful.

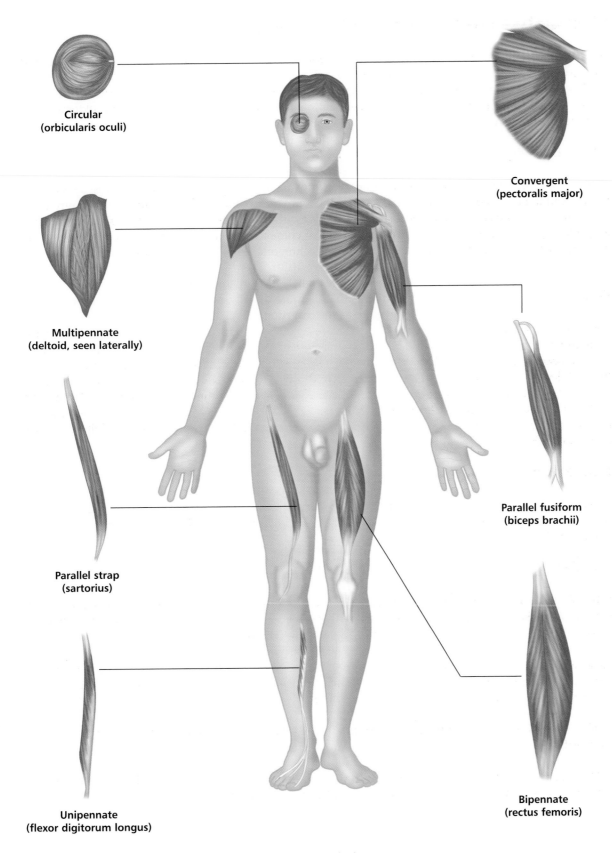

Circular
(orbicularis oculi)

Convergent
(pectoralis major)

Multipennate
(deltoid, seen laterally)

Parallel fusiform
(biceps brachii)

Parallel strap
(sartorius)

Unipennate
(flexor digitorum longus)

Bipennate
(rectus femoris)

Figure 1.30: Muscle shapes.

Musculo-skeletal Mechanics

Origins and Insertions

In the majority of movements, one attachment of a muscle remains relatively stationary while the attachment at the other end moves. The more stationary attachment is called the *origin* of the muscle, and the other attachment is called the *insertion*. A spring that closes a gate could be said to have its origin on the gate-post and its insertion on the gate itself. In the body, the arrangement is rarely so clear-cut, because depending on the activity one is engaged in, the fixed and moveable ends of the muscle may be reversed. For example, muscles that attach the upper limb to the chest normally move the arm relative to the trunk; which means their origins are on the trunk and their insertions are on the upper limb. However, in climbing, the arms are fixed, while the trunk is moved as it is pulled up to the fixed limbs. In this type of situation, where the insertion is fixed and the origin moves, the muscle is said to perform a *reversed action*. Because there are so many situations where muscles are working with a reversed action, it is sometimes less confusing to simply speak of 'attachments', without reference to origin and insertion.

In practice, muscle attachments that lie more proximally, i.e. more towards the trunk or on the trunk, are usually referred to as the origin. Attachments that lie more distally, i.e. away from the attached end of a limb, or away from the trunk, are referred to as the insertion.

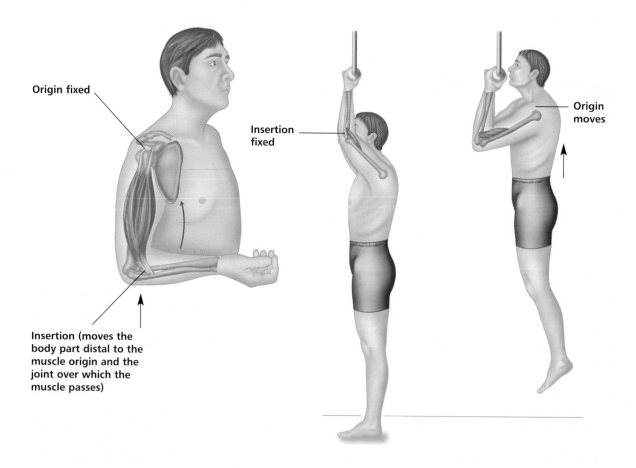

Figure 1.31: Muscle working with origin fixed and insertion moving.

Figure 1.32: Climbing: muscles are working with insertion fixed and origin moving (reversed action).

Group Action of Muscles

Muscles work together, or in opposition, to achieve a wide variety of movements. Therefore, whatever one muscle can do, there is another muscle that can undo it. Muscles may also be required to provide additional support or stability to enable certain movements to occur elsewhere. Muscles are classified into four functional groups:

- Prime Mover or Agonist
- Antagonist
- Synergist
- Fixator

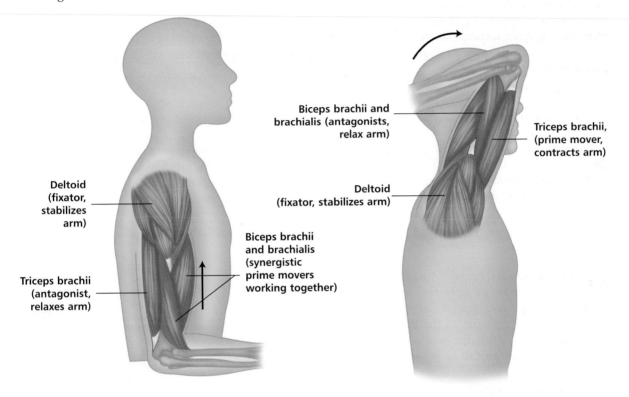

Figure 1.33: Group action of muscles; a) flexing arm at elbow, b) extending arm at elbow
(showing reversed roles of prime mover and anatagonist).

Prime Mover or Agonist

A *prime mover* (also called an *agonist*) is a muscle that contracts to produce a specified movement. An example is the biceps brachii, which is the prime mover of elbow flexion. Other muscles may assist the prime mover in providing the same movement, albeit with less effect. Such muscles are called *assistant* or *secondary movers*. For example, the brachialis assists the biceps brachii in flexing the elbow, and is therefore a secondary mover.

Antagonist

The muscle on the opposite side of a joint to the prime mover, and which must relax to allow the prime mover to contract, is called an *antagonist*. For example, when the biceps brachii on the front of the arm contract to flex the elbow, the triceps brachii on the back of the arm must relax to allow this movement to occur. When the movement is reversed, i.e. when the elbow is extended, the triceps brachii becomes the *prime mover* and the biceps brachii assumes the role of *antagonist*.

Synergist

Synergists prevent any unwanted movements that might occur as the prime mover contracts. This is especially important where a prime mover crosses two joints, because when it contracts it will cause movement at both joints, unless other muscles act to stabilize one of the joints. For example, the muscles that flex the fingers not only cross the finger joints, but also cross the wrist joint, potentially causing movement at both joints. However, it is because you have other muscles acting synergistically to stabilize the wrist joint that you are able to flex the fingers into a fist without also flexing the wrist at the same time.

A prime mover may have more than one action, so synergists also act to eliminate the unwanted movements. For example, the biceps brachii will flex the elbow, but its line of pull will also supinate the forearm (twist the forearm, as in tightening a screw). If you want flexion to occur without supination, other muscles must contract to prevent this supination. In this context, such synergists are sometimes called *neutralisers*.

Fixator

A synergist is more specifically referred to as a fixator or stabilizer when it immobilizes the bone of the prime mover's origin, thus providing a stable base for the action of the prime mover. The muscles that stabilize (fix) the scapula during movements of the upper limb are good examples. The sit-up exercise gives another good example: The abdominal muscles attach to both the ribcage and the pelvis. When they contract to enable you to perform a sit-up, the hip flexors will contract synergistically as fixators to prevent the abdominals tilting the pelvis; enabling the upper body to curl forward as the pelvis remains stationary.

Leverage

The bones, joints, and muscles together form a system of levers in the body, in order to optimise the relative strength, range and speed required of any given movement. The joints act as the fulcra (**sing**. fulcrum), while the muscles apply the effort and the bones bear the weight of the body part to be moved.

A muscle attached close to the fulcrum will be relatively weaker than it would be if it were attached further away. However, it is able to produce a greater range and speed of movement; because the length of the lever amplifies the distance travelled by its moveable attachment. Figure 1.34 illustrates this in relation to the adductors of the hip joint. The muscle so positioned to move the greater load (in this case, adductor longus) is said to have a *mechanical advantage*. The muscle attached close to the fulcra is said to operate at a *mechanical disadvantage*, although it can move a load more rapidly through larger distances.

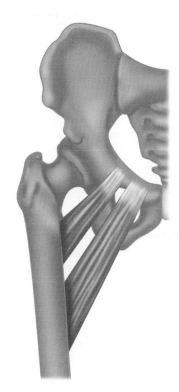

Figure 1.34: The pectineus is attached closer to the axis of movement than the adductor longus. Therefore, the pectineus is the weaker adductor of the hip, but is able to produce a greater movement of the lower limb per centimetre of contraction.

The following illustrations depict the differences in first, second and third class levers, with examples in the human body.

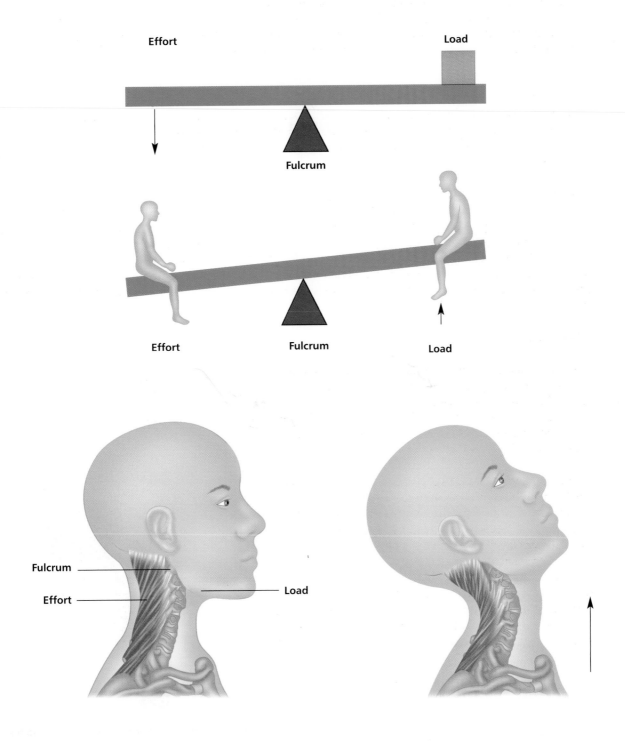

Figure 1.35: First-class lever: The relative position of components is Load-Fulcrum-Effort. Examples include a seesaw (as above). Another example is a pair of scissors. In the body, an example is the ability to extend the head and neck, i.e. the facial structures are the load; the atlanto-occipital joint is the fulcrum; the posterior neck muscles provide the effort.

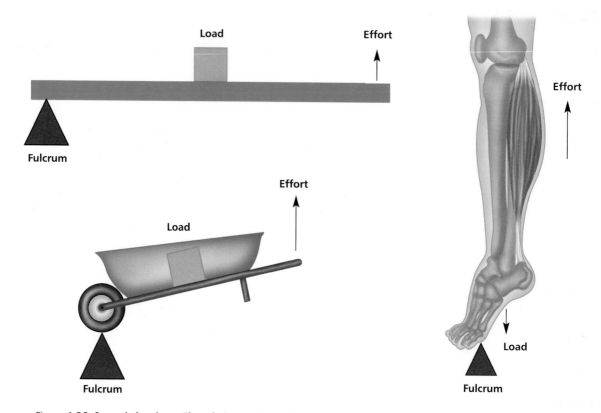

Figure 1.36: Second-class lever: The relative position of components is Fulcrum-Load-Effort. The best example is a wheelbarrow. In the body, an example is the ability to raise the heels off the ground in standing, i.e. the ball of the foot is the fulcrum; the body-weight is the load; the calf muscles provide the effort. With second-class levers, speed and range of movement are sacrificed for strength.

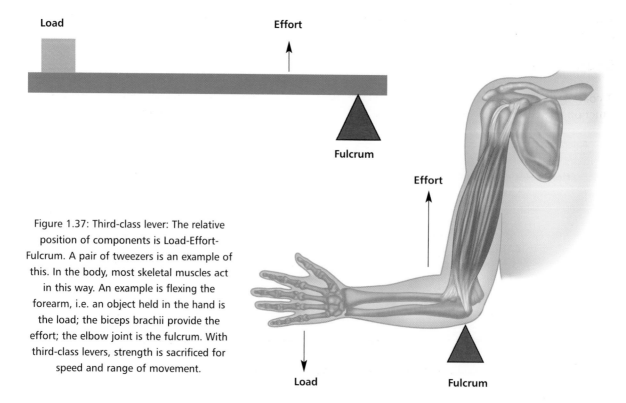

Figure 1.37: Third-class lever: The relative position of components is Load-Effort-Fulcrum. A pair of tweezers is an example of this. In the body, most skeletal muscles act in this way. An example is flexing the forearm, i.e. an object held in the hand is the load; the biceps brachii provide the effort; the elbow joint is the fulcrum. With third-class levers, strength is sacrificed for speed and range of movement.

Fascia and Myofascia

It is worth spending some time exploring this tissue, since it is directly implicated in the manifestation of trigger points.

Myofascia

The superficial fascia which invests muscle is also known as *connective tissue*. It is a clear, fibrous tissue. It is modified according to where it is located in the body (*superficial* or *deep*) but it is somewhat like 'cling-film' in nature. For example, if you eat chicken, you may well be aware of the superficial fascia; this lies under the skin and is a tough, transparent (cling-film like) tissue layer. This myofascia invests muscles like an envelope. It is plastic-like; when it is injured or damaged, it becomes shorter, condensed, and tighter. Trigger points mainly manifest in the myofascial tissue; the contracture of this fascia gives rise to nodules underneath the skin. Depending on where it is located, it is classified in many different ways:

Endomysium

A delicate connective tissue called *endomysium* lies outside the sarcolemma of each muscle fibre, separating each fibre from its neighbours, but also connecting them together.

Fasciculi

Muscle fibres are arranged in parallel bundles called *fasciculi*.

Perimysium

Each fasciculus is bound by a denser collagenic sheath called the *perimysium*.

Epimysium

The entire muscle, which is therefore an assembly of fasciculi, is wrapped in a fibrous sheath called the *epimysium*.

Deep Fascia

A coarser sheet of fibrous connective tissue lies outside the epimysium, binding individual muscles into functional groups. This deep fascia extends to wrap around other adjacent structures.

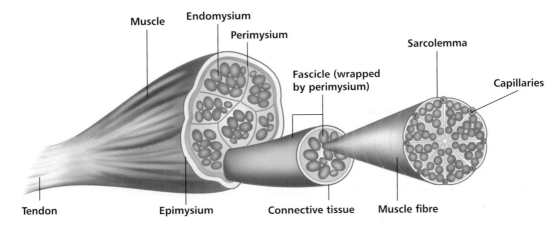

Figure 1.38: The connective tissue sheaths of skeletal muscle.

Muscle Attachment

The way a muscle attaches to bone or other tissues is either through a direct attachment or an indirect attachment. A direct attachment (called a *fleshy attachment*) is where the perimysium and epimysium of the muscle unite and fuse with the periosteum of a bone, perichondrium of a cartilage, a joint capsule, or the connective tissue underlying the skin (some muscles of facial expression being good examples of the latter). An indirect attachment is where the connective tissue components of a muscle fuse together into bundles of collagen fibres to form an intervening tendon. Indirect attachments are much more common. The types of tendinous attachments are as follows:

Tendons and Aponeurosis

Muscle fascia, which is the connective tissue component of a muscle, combine together and extend beyond the end of the muscle as round cords or flat bands, called *tendons*; or as a thin, flat and broad *aponeurosis*. The tendon or aponeurosis secures the muscle to the bone or cartilage, to the fascia of other muscles, or to a seam of fibrous tissue called a *raphe*. Flat patches of tendon may form on the body of a muscle where it is exposed to friction. For example, on the deep surface of trapezius, where it rubs against the spine of the scapula.

Intermuscular Septa

In some cases, flat sheets of dense connective tissue known as *intermuscular septa* penetrate between muscles, providing another medium to which muscle fibres may attach.

Sesamoid Bones

If a tendon is subject to friction, it may, but not necessarily, develop a *sesamoid bone* within its substance. An example is the peroneus longus tendon in the sole of the foot. However, sesamoid bones may also appear in tendons not subject to friction.

Multiple Attachments

Many muscles have only two attachments, one at each end. However, more complex muscles are often attached to several different structures at its origin and/or its insertion. If these attachments are separated, effectively meaning the muscle gives rise to two or more tendons and/or aponeurosis inserting into different places, the muscle is said to have two heads. For example, the biceps brachii has two heads at its origin; one from the corocoid process of the scapula and one the other from the supraglenoid tubercle. The triceps brachii has three heads and the quadriceps has four.

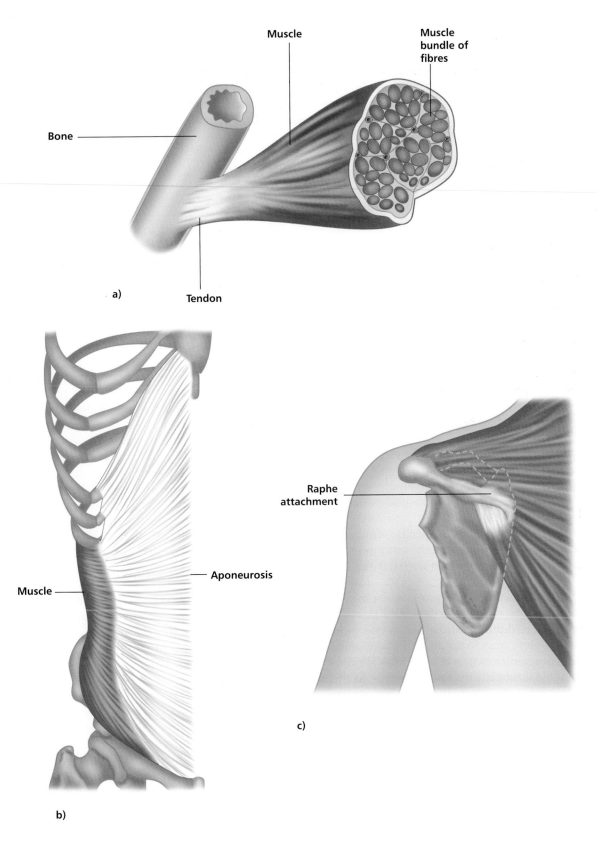

Figure 1.39: a) a tendon attachment; b) an attachment by aponeurosis;
c) flat patches of tendon on the deep surface of trapezius (raphe attachment).

Myofascial and Embryological Development

An overview of the embryological origin of connective tissues may provide some insights into the formation and location of trigger points. Trigger points tend to manifest within the *epimysium* according to myofascial strain patterns. These patterns start to develop very early on, both in the developing embryo and may also be related to foetal alignment in the womb. These strain patterns develop as we mature from childhood to adulthood and are influenced by, for example, posture, weight gain, and mechanical injury (*see* page 48).

Embryological Development of Fascia

As stated above, fascia supports organs, wraps around muscles, and condenses to form ligaments, aponeuroses and even bones.

By the end of the seventh week of development, the embryo has most of its organs, bones, muscles, and neurovascular structures in place. Around these primitive structures, a group of 'filler cells' begin to proliferate. This filler is derived from *mesodermal tissue*, a primitive fascia that is constructed from cells, fibres, and intercellular matrix. This matrix has the consistency of glass wool in a soft, jelly-like substrate. In most body areas, this primitive fascia remains supple until birth. In some areas however, it condenses and becomes 'directional', in response to internal and external pressures and tensions. Ligaments and tendons begin to form in these areas. Stress and strain lines develop in these tissues, and bone salts are laid-down, causing primitive ossification. As the bones grow, they drag some of the primitive connective tissue fibres into 'differentiated' ligaments. An example of this is the pre-vertebral cartilage, which grows and pushes into the mesodermal connective tissue beds. As it does so, it creates lines of stress that help to maintain integrity and provide a scaffold for further directional growth. As the bones start to grow, the complexity of strains and directional pulls results in the differentiated spinal ligaments (flavum, posterior longitudinal, etc.).

Furthermore, it has been reliably demonstrated that primitive organ growth relies on this mesodermal intracellular matrix. The 'potential' pancreas for example will only differentiate into a mature organ in the specific presence of this 'primitive' potential fascia. It has been suggested that the primitive or potential fascia creates a 'specific energy field' in which the cells of the 'potential' organ mature and differentiate.[19] This may make more sense when we consider that the bones, muscles, ligaments, and myofascial elements of connective tissue all share a characteristic pattern of growth.

The relationship between a developing muscle and its enveloping connective tissue myofascia is complex. The stress lines, described above may provide a key to understanding this relationship. It has been suggested that during the second month of embryological development, connective tissue is laid down before muscle tissue, and that clumps of 'potential muscle tissue, caught within this directional pull, differentiates into mature muscle oriented along the line of pull'.[19] These clumps of muscle tissue elongate through directional pressure. At this point they develop, differentiate, mature and grow in size through mitotic cell reproduction to form the muscles as we know them.

In other words, it is the growth of fascia along lines of stress and strain that is the powerhouse of muscle orientation and development. This also explains why muscle action is not singular, but interconnected. For example, a contraction of the biceps brachii muscle will exert a force on the fascia of the whole arm, shoulder, and neck. Fascia has no beginning or end and is described by anatomists according to location. On closer inspection the myofascial bags surrounding the muscles are actually part of a continuum. This may also go some way to explaining the referred pain patterns stimulated by pressing on a trigger point.

2

An Overview of Trigger Points

Definition

"A highly irritable localized spot of exquisite tenderness in a nodule in a palpable taught band of (skeletal) muscle."
(Travell & Simons, 1993).

These 'spots' can range in size from a 'tiny lump' to 'little peas' to 'large lumps', and can be felt beneath the surface embedded within the muscle fibres. If they are tender to pressure they may well be 'trigger points'. The size of a trigger point nodule varies according to the size, shape, and type of muscle in which it is generated. What is consistent is that they are tender to pressure. So tender in fact that when they are pressed, the patient often winces from the pain; this has been called the *'jump sign'*.

Prevalence

Myofascial trigger points may well be implicated in all types of musculo-skeletal and mechanical muscular pain. Their presence has even been demonstrated in children and babies. Pain or symptoms may be directly due to active trigger points or pain may 'build-up' over time from latent or inactive trigger points. Studies and investigations in selected patient populations have been carried out on various regions of the body. These have confirmed a high prevalence of trigger point pain. The following table lists some of these studies.[25]

Body region	Research centre	Population	% with myofascial pain
General	Medical[22]	172 (54)	30
General	Pain Medicine Center[10]	96	93
General	Comprehensive Pain Center[6]	283	85
Craniofacial	Head & Neck Pain Clinic[8]	164	55
Lumbogluteal	Orthopaedic Clinic[9]	97	21

Table 1: Prevalence of trigger points in selected patient populations.

There is a large body of research evidence directly linking musculo-skeletal pain to trigger points.

Embryogenesis

There is some evidence that myofascial trigger points may be present in babies and children.[3] They have also been demonstrated in muscle tissue after death!

Trigger points develop in the myofascia, mainly in the centre of the muscle belly where the motor end plate enters (primary or central). However, secondary or satellite trigger points often develop in a response to the primary trigger point. These satellite points often develop along fascial lines of stress. As described above, these lines of stress may well be 'built-in' at the time of embryogenesis. External factors such as ageing, body morphology, posture, weight gain or congenital malformation, etc., also play a crucial part in trigger point manifestation and genesis (*see* page 48).

Evidence

In 1957, Dr. Janet Travell discovered that trigger points 'generate and receive' minute electrical currents. She determined experimentally that trigger point activity could be accurately quantified by measuring these signals with an electromyogram (EMG). She went on to demonstrate that a trigger point could be accurately and reliably located by the same technique. This is due to the fact that in its resting state, electrical activity in muscles is 'silent'. When a small part of the muscle goes into contracture, as is the case with a trigger point, it causes a small localized spike in electrical activity.

More easily, trigger points can be palpated beneath the skin in specific locations. They are *localized, nodular* and *discrete* and are characteristically painful, producing reproducible patterns of referred pain.

Acupuncture or Acupressure Points and Trigger Points

Whilst there may be some overlap in trigger points and acupuncture points, they are not equivalent. Acupuncture points are said to be localized concentrations of 'energy' which develop along electromagnetic lines (meridians). Trigger points on the other hand are discreet nodular tetherings in the myofascial tissues, which when stimulated cause a specific and reproducible referred pain pattern.

Based on the above theory of the 'specific energy field' generated by fascia, it may be that myofascial trigger points develop along lines of altered energetic activity or at the very least altered strain patterns. Some authorities go much further, claiming that there is a 70% correlation between trigger points and acupuncture points.[2] It has been suggested that the general theory of acupuncture points may have been put forward by ancient Chinese medicine as an 'explanation' for the demonstrable and palpable presence of trigger points within myofascial tissues.[25] Furthermore, there is some evidence to demonstrate increased efficacy in pain relief, when the trigger point is present at the site of an acupuncture point during treatment.[17]

Fibromyalgia

Fibromyalgia syndrome is characterized by widespread diffuse musculo-skeletal pain and fatigue. It is a disorder for which the cause is still unknown. *Fibromyalgia means pain in the fibrous, connective and tendinous tissues of the body. 'Fibromyalgia is a complex syndrome characterized by pain amplification, musculo-skeletal discomfort, and systemic symptoms'.*[24] It has now been 'firmly established' that a central nervous system (CNS) dysfunction is primarily responsible for this amplification in the pain pathway.

Like myofascial trigger points, pain arises from the connective tissues, muscles, tendons, and ligaments. Similarly, fibromyalgia does not involve the joints. Both conditions are often mistaken; however, they are discreet conditions. Both conditions may be linked to psychological depression. Unlike trigger point manifestation, fibromyalgia is believed to stem from a systemic origin.

Unlike trigger points, which cause a specific and reproducible pattern of referral, patients with fibromyalgia describe that they *ache all over* (although some do describe localized tender spots). Patients with fibromyalgia describe their muscles as feeling like they have been pulled or overworked. Sometimes the muscles twitch and at other times they burn. More women than men are affected by fibromyalgia, but there is no age profile. Unlike fibromyalgia points, trigger points have been successfully photographed using electron microscopy. A table listing the basic differences is listed overleaf.

	Pain location	Type of pain	Muscular quality on palpation
Trigger point	Specific & discrete	Referred in a specific pattern	Tight & stiff, warm
Fibromyalgia	General	Vague, aching, burning, diffuse, widespread	Doughy & soft

Table 2: Some basic differences between fibromyalgia and trigger points.[14]

Add to this list that in fibromyalgia the pain is mediated centrally (CNS) and for trigger points, pain is mediated locally in the region of the motor end plate from the peripheral nervous system (PNS).

3

Physiology of Trigger Points

Skeletal (somatic or voluntary) muscles make up approximately 40% of the total human body weight. Several theories have been advanced for how trigger points develop within muscles. I will be presenting the most widely accepted hypothesis. In order to understand how a trigger point develops, it is useful for us to review the physiological mechanism of muscle contraction.

The primary function of skeletal (somatic or voluntary) muscles is to produce movement through the ability to contract and relax in a coordinated manner. They are attached to bone by tendons. The place where a muscle attaches to a relatively stationary point on a bone, either directly or via a tendon, is called the *origin*. When the muscle contracts, it transmits tension to the bones across one or more joints, and movement occurs. The end of the muscle that attaches to the bone that moves is called the *insertion*.

Overview of Skeletal Muscle Structure

The functional unit of skeletal muscle is known as a *muscle fibre,* which is an elongated, cylindrical cell with multiple nuclei, ranging from 10 to 100 microns in width, and a few millimetres to 30+ centimetres in length. The cytoplasm of the fibre is called the *sarcoplasm,* which is encapsulated inside a cell membrane called the *sarcolemma.* A delicate membrane known as the *endomysium* surrounds each individual fibre.

These fibres are grouped together in bundles covered by the *perimysium.* These bundles are themselves grouped together, and the whole muscle is encased in a sheath called the *epimysium.* These muscle membranes lie through the entire length of the muscle, from the tendon of origin to the tendon of insertion. This whole structure is sometimes referred to as the *musculo-tendinous unit.*

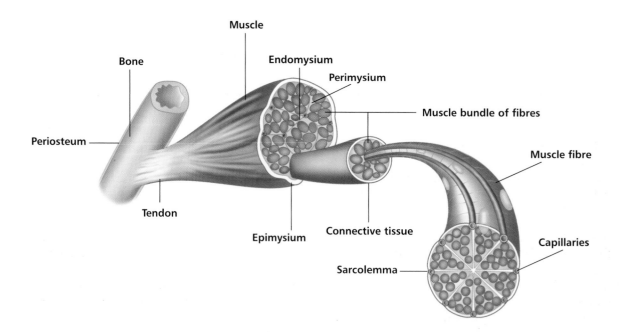

Figure 3.1: Cross-section of muscle tissue.

The active component of muscle activity occurs at the microscopic level; at the level of the *myofibril.*

Myofibrils

Through an electron microscope, one can distinguish the contractile elements of a muscle fibre, known as *myofibrils*, running the whole length of the fibre. Each myofibril reveals alternate light and dark banding, producing the characteristic cross-striation of the muscle fibre. These bands are called *myofilaments*. The light bands are referred to as isotropic (I) bands, and consist of thin myofilaments made of the protein *actin*. The dark one's are called anisotropic (A) bands, consisting of thicker myofilaments made of the protein *myosin*. (Note that a third connecting filament made of a protein called *titin* is now recognized). The myosin filaments have paddle-like extensions that emanate from the filaments rather like the oars of a boat. These extensions latch on to the actin filaments, forming what are described as 'cross-bridges' between the two types of filaments. The cross-bridges, using the energy of ATP, pull the actin strands closer together*. Thus, the light and dark sets of filaments increasingly overlap, like the interlocking of fingers, resulting in muscle contraction. One set of actin-myosin filaments is called a *sarcomere*.

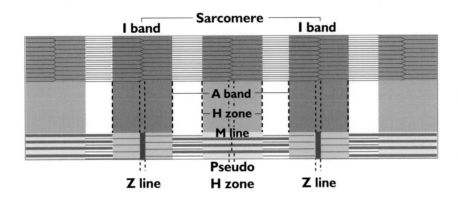

Figure 3.2: The myofilaments in a sarcomere. A sarcomere is bounded at both ends by the Z line.

- The lighter zone is known as the I band, and the darker zone the A band.
- The Z line is a thin dark line at the midpoint of the I band.
- A sarcomere is defined as the section of myofibril between one Z line and the next.
- The centre of the A band contains the H zone.
- The M line bisects the H zone, and delineates the centre of the sarcomere.

If an outside force causes a muscle to stretch beyond its resting level of tonus, the interlinking effect of the actin and myosin filaments that occurs during contraction is reversed. Initially, the actin and myosin filaments accommodate the stretch, but as the stretch continues, the titin filaments increasingly 'pay out' to absorb the displacement. Thus, it is the titin filament that determines the muscle fibre's extensibility and resistance to stretch. Research indicates that a muscle fibre (sarcomere), if properly prepared, can be elongated up to 150% of its normal length at rest.

---

* Huxley's Sliding Filament Theory
The generally accepted hypothesis to explain muscle function is partly described by Huxley's sliding filament theory (Huxley and Hanson, 1954). Muscle fibres receive a nerve impulse that cause the release of calcium ions stored in the muscle. In the presence of the muscles fuel, known as adenosine triphosphate (ATP), the calcium ions bind with the actin and myosin filaments to form an electrostatic (magnetic) bond. This bond causes the fibres to shorten, resulting in their contraction or increase in tonus. When the nerve impulse ceases, the muscle fibres relax. Their elastic elements recoil the filaments to their non-contracted lengths, i.e. their resting level of tonus.

Trigger Points Within Sarcomeres

Muscle contraction occurs at the level of the sarcomeres. Even the slightest of *gross movements* requires the co-ordinated contraction of millions of sarcomeres. The sliding process (above) requires: a) an initializing stimulation or impulse from a local motor nerve; b) energy, and c) calcium ions.

Physiology of Movement

When the brain wants to move a muscle, it fires a message through a motor nerve. The local motor nerve terminals translate this impulse chemically by producing acetylcholine (ACh). ACh triggers an increase in sarcomere activity. The energy required for this process is released by the mitochondria (energy centres) in the cells. Calcium ions inhabit the sarcoplasmic reticulum, which is found in the sarcoplasm of skeletal muscle.

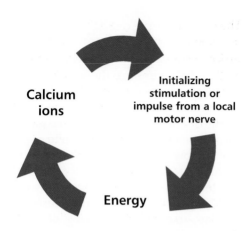

Figure 3.3: Flow chart for nerve impulse to cause muscle contraction.

Trigger Point Development

Trigger points manifest where sarcomeres become over-active. We are still not 100% sure what causes this to happen. It is probably multifactorial. Hypotheses include:

- Increased acetylcholine production;
- Changes in calcium metabolism – excess calcium release;
- Hypertension;
- Stress;
- Localized neurological hyper-stimulation;
- Other.

Whatever the stimulus, the actin and myosin myofilaments stop sliding over one another. As a result, the sarcomere becomes turned to the permanently '*switched-on*' position leading to a contraction. This sustained sarcomere contraction leads to local intracellular chemical changes including:

- Localized ischemia;
- Increased metabolism needs;
- Increased energy required to sustain contraction;
- Failed re-uptake of calcium ions into the sarcoplasmic reticulum;
- Localized inflammation (to facilitate repair);
- Compression / watershed effect on local vessels;
- Energy crisis;
- Increased production of inflammatory agents which sensitize local autonomic and nociceptive (pain) fibres.

If this situation is allowed to persist over a significant period of time, the above changes lead to a *vicious cycle*. Calcium is unable to be taken into the actin and myosin myofilaments leading to sarcomere 'failure'.

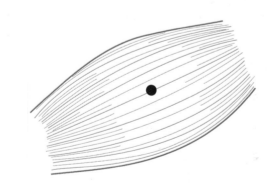

Figure 3.4: A trigger point (*the blue dot is to be used in Chapters 5–10 to indicate the location of a trigger point. Remember, it is not always at this point, *see* page 7).

The body attempts to resolve this situation by changing the blood supply to the sarcomere (vasodilation). One further result of this anomalous situation is the migration of localized *acute* and *chronic* inflammatory cells. Inflammation is a cascade; this cascade mechanism starts to occur around the *dysfunctional* sarcomere. Inflammation brings with it sensitizing substances such as substance P, a peptide which, for example, increases the contraction of gastrointestinal smooth muscle, and causes further vasodilation. This has the effect of stimulating both local (small) pain fibres and local autonomic fibres. This in turn leads to increased acetylcholine production and hence a vicious cycle.

Eventually the brain sends a signal to rest the muscle in which the trigger point manifests. This also leads to muscle hypertonia, weakness, shortening, and fibrosis (muscle stiffness). Treatment is thus aimed at disrupting and attenuating this vicious cycle.

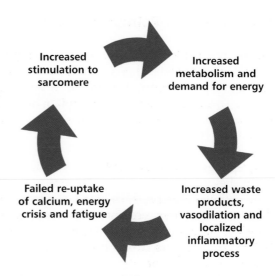

Increased stimulation to sarcomere

Increased metabolism and demand for energy

Increased waste products, vasodilation and localized inflammatory process

Failed re-uptake of calcium, energy crisis and fatigue

Figure 3.5: Vicious cycle for trigger point physiology.

Trigger Point Classification

Trigger points are described in various ways according to location, tenderness and chronicity: central (or primary); satellite (or secondary); attachment; diffuse; inactive (or latent); and active.

Central (or Primary) Trigger Points

These are the most well-established and 'florid' when they are *active*, and are usually what people refer to when they talk about trigger points. The central trigger points always exist in the centre of the muscle belly; this is where the motor end plate enters the muscle. N.B. Muscle shape and fibre arrangement is of importance in this regard. For example, in multipennate muscles, there may be *several* central points. Also, if muscle fibres run diagonally, this may lead to variations in trigger point location.

Satellite (or Secondary) Trigger Points

Trigger points may be 'created' as a response to the central trigger point in neighbouring muscles that lie within the *referred pain zone*. In such cases, the primary trigger point is still the key to therapeutic intervention and the satellite trigger points often resolve once the primary point has been effectively rendered inactive. The corollary is also true in that satellite points may prove resilient to treatment until the primary central focus is weakened; such is often the case in the para-spinal and / or abdominal muscles.

Attachment Trigger Points

Myofascia is a continuum, as discussed earlier (*see* page 33). It has been noted that the area where the tendon inserts into the bone (tendino-osseous) is often 'exquisitely' tender.[25, 3] This may well be the result of the existing forces travelling across these regions. It has been also suggested (ibid) that this may result from an associated chronic, active myofascial trigger point. This is because the tenderness has been demonstrated to reduce once the primary central trigger point has been treated; in such cases, the point is described as an attachment trigger point. Furthermore, it has been suggested that if a chronic situation occurs where the primary and attachment trigger points remain untreated, 'degenerative changes' within the joint may be precipitated and accelerated.[25]

Diffuse Trigger Points

Trigger points can sometimes occur where multiple satellite trigger points exist secondary to multiple central trigger points. This is often the case when there is a severe postural deformity such as a scoliosis, and an entire quadrant of the body is involved. In this scenario the secondary points are said to be *diffuse*. These diffuse trigger points often develop along lines of altered *stress* and / or *strain* patterns.

Inactive (or Latent) Trigger Points

This applies to lumps and nodules which feel like trigger points. These can develop anywhere in the body; they are often secondary. These trigger points are not however painful, and do not elicit a referred pain pathway. The presence of inactive trigger points within muscles may lead to increased muscular *stiffness*. It has been suggested that these points are more common in those who live a sedentary lifestyle.[24] It is also worth noting here that these points may re-activate if the central or primary trigger point is (re-)stimulated, or following trauma and injury.

Active Trigger Points

This can apply to central or satellite trigger points. A variety of stimulants can activate an inactive trigger point such as forcing muscular activity through pain. This situation is common when increasing activity post road traffic accident (RTA) where multiple and diffuse trigger points may have developed. The term denotes that the trigger point is both tender to palpation and elicits a referred pain pattern.

Trigger Point Symptoms

Referred Pain Patterns

Pain is a complex symptom experienced differently and individually. However, referred pain is the *defining symptom* of a myofascial trigger point.

You may be used to the idea of referred pain of a visceral origin; an example of this is heart pain. A myocardial infarct (heart attack) is often not experienced as crushing chest pain, but as pain in the left arm and hand, and the left jaw. This type of pain is well-documented and known to originate from the embryological dermomyotome; in this case, the heart tissue, jaw tissue, and arm tissues all develop from the same dermomyotome.

Referred pain from a myofascial trigger point is somewhat different. It is a distinct and discreet pattern or map of pain. This map is consistent and has no racial or gender differences. The pain is generated by stimulating an active trigger point.

Patients describe referred pain in this map as having a *deep, aching* quality; movement may sometimes exacerbate symptoms making the pain *sharper*. An example of this might be a headache. The patient often describes a pattern of pain, or ache, which can sometimes be aggravated and made sharper by moving the head and neck. The intensity of pain will vary according to the following factors (this list is not exhaustive):

• Location (attachment points are more sensitive);
• Degree of trigger point irritability;
• Active or latent trigger points;
• Primary or satellite trigger points;
• Site of trigger point (some areas are more sensitive);
• Associated tissue damage;

- Location / host tissue stiffness or flexibility;
- Ageing;
- Chronicity of trigger point.

Autonomic Effects

The nervous system is divided into central (CNS), peripheral (PNS) and autonomic (ANS). The autonomic nervous system is responsible for regulating many of our *automatic* or *vegetative* functions such as sweating and digestion. From our discussion on the physiology of trigger points, it can be seen that autonomic nerve fibres are implicated in the pathogenesis of a trigger point. Therapeutic treatment of myofascial trigger points has been demonstrated to have an effect on the ANS.[25]

Physical Findings

The language for describing sensation is not a highly sophisticated one. Unfortunately we have not yet evolved a suitable language to classify what we feel with our hands. With this in mind I will attempt to classify how trigger points feel.

- Small nodules the size of a pinhead;
- Pea sized nodules;
- Large lumps;
- Several large lumps next to each other;
- Tender spots embedded in taut bands of semi-hard muscle that feels like a cord;
- Rope-like bands lying next to each other like partially cooked spaghetti;
- The skin over a trigger point is often slightly warmer than the surrounding skin due to increased metabolic / autonomic activity.

Known symptoms include:

Autonomic changes
- Hypersalivation – increased saliva;
- Epiphora – abnormal overflow of tears down the cheek;
- Conjunctivitis – reddening of the eyes;
- Ptosis – drooping of the eyelids;
- Blurring of vision;
- Increased nasal secretion;
- Goose bumps.

Examination

Examination may be performed standing, sitting, or lying down. The choice depends on both the area being examined and the type of muscle fibre suspected. You may want to examine a muscle *under load* if you suspect this is an aggravating factor.

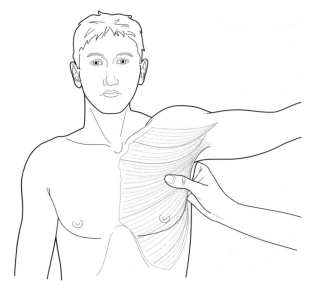

Figure 3.6: Pectoralis major examination.

For simplicity, *from this point forward*, I will describe the examination of the pectoralis major and its trigger point(s).

The main trigger points in the pectoralis major are to be found in the clavicular portion of the muscle. A *pincer* like grip is the best way of examining for a trigger point in this region. Trigger points in the parasternal region of the muscle are best palpated with a flat-handed contact.

Procedure:

- With the patient sitting or standing;
- Patient asked to abduct the arm 90° to put the muscle into moderate tension;
- Palpate for nodule or tight band;
- Feel for the *jump sign* or *twitch* response;
- Pressure should reproduce symptoms experienced by the patient;
- Pressure should elicit a referred pain pattern.

Maintaining Factors

The following are maintaining factors for trigger points. The presence of one or several of these may well present some difficulty in eliminating trigger points over the long-term.

- Ageing;
- Posture (including work);
- Obesity;
- Anorexia;
- Scar tissue (post surgical);
- Sports, hobbies, habits;
- Stress and strain patterns;
- Metabolic disorders;
- Disease or illness;
- Vitamin deficiency;
- Congenital (bony) anomaly;
- Type of muscle fibre;
- Direction / orientation of muscle fibre;
- Muscle shape / morphology (fusiform, etc.);
- Psychological factors;
- Chronicity of trigger point.

Advice to Patient

Once a therapeutic intervention has been performed, it is advisable to encourage the patient to get involved in managing their own symptoms. In this book, I have offered some specific advice under the

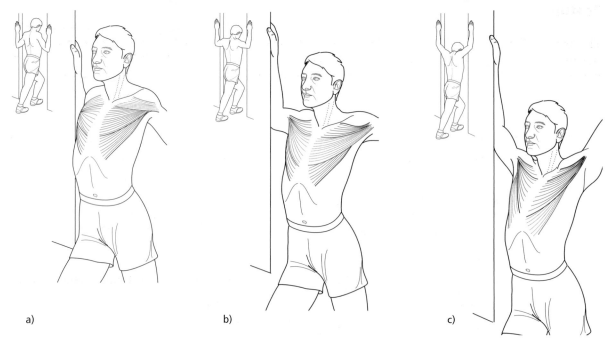

a)   b)   c)

Figure 3.7: Stretching techniques for pectoralis major; a) upper fibres, b) middle fibres, c) lower fibres.

heading 'advice to patient'. As a more general overview, you might want to include hints, tips, and advice using the following elements or components.

By way of an example, I will use the pectoralis major muscle again.

Strengthening

Where muscles are weak, they may be more susceptible to damage, fatigue and injury. Weakness is often a contributory factor in the pathogenesis of myofascial trigger points. This is because the body overcompensates for the weakness and strains in the muscle – overloading and overstimulating the motor end plate. I have illustrated some simple strengthening diagrams where appropriate.

One muscle should never be strengthened in isolation. If you decide to offer strengthening exercises, it is advisable to put them in context. An overall stretching programme should be advised, perhaps utilizing a yoga-based regime.

Stretching

I have illustrated some simple stretching diagrams where appropriate. Stretching should be performed slowly, and *without* bouncing. Care must be taken to isolate the stretch to the specific muscle as far as possible. As a rule, stretches should be performed three times, slightly deepening the stretch with an out-breath each time. This sequence should be performed several times per day, for approximately 15–20 minutes.

Advice

Most of the advice you can offer is common sense. *"Look at your driving position"*, *"Look at your every day work set-up"*. In the example of the pectoralis major muscle you may ask the patient about their stress or anxiety levels (rib breathing mechanics). If your patient has large, heavy breasts, you may want to advise on a more appropriate bra or support. I have tried to offer some advice for each muscle in this book.

Posture

This may well have a crucial role in maintaining trigger point activity. Faulty sitting and / or standing postures are both a pathogenic and maintaining factor for trigger point activity. Advice and exercises for posture is often the key to unlocking both *central* and *satellite* points.

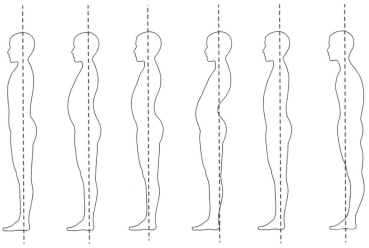

Figure 3.8: Posture.

Sleeping Posture

Patients often assume strange postures at night! This is sometimes to reduce the pain from either active, or stiff latent trigger points; in such cases patients often opt for a sleeping position which shortens the affected muscle. For example, sleeping with either the hands above the head (supraspinatus), or the arms folded over the chest (pectoralis major). In other cases, it may be that the sleeping position is a pathogenic or a maintaining factor.

Work Posture

Some patients may have manual or repetitive working activities; these may well have a role to play in trigger point pathogenesis or maintenance. Many patients spend their time at work sitting. Below is a diagram illustrating an ideal sitting work posture.

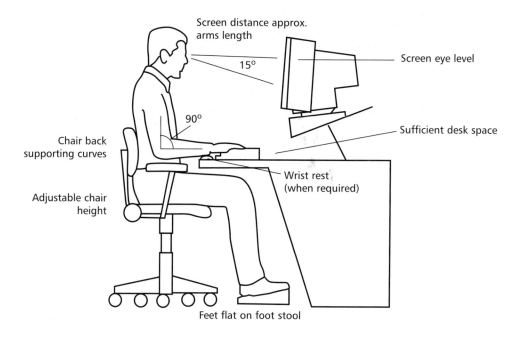

Figure 3.9: Ideal sitting work posture.

Habitual Activity, Hobbies, and Sports

Similarly, it is important to ask the patient if they perform any repetitive or habitual activities. Standing all day on one leg, for example may well overload the tensor fasciae latae (TFL) muscle. Sitting in a cross-legged position may affect a range of muscles such as the hip flexors (iliopsoas), the buttock muscles (gluteals and piriformis) and the thigh muscles (quadriceps). Heavy smokers may develop trigger points in the shoulder (deltoid) and arm (biceps) muscles.

Similarly, certain hobbies and sports may lead to an increased incidence of trigger point pathogenesis. It is important to ask carefully about such activities. What is the level of competence? Does the patient warm up, and warm down? How competitive are they? Is their level of activity realistic for their age? Posture? Body type? Physical health? You may want to explore these areas further. It is often useful to run through these activities and set the patient certain activity goals to achieve in between treatment sessions.

4

Therapeutic Technique Protocols

Palpation

Palpation is as much an art as it is a science. Initially you should seek to relax the patient sufficiently to gain access to vulnerable and potentially painful treatment. A thorough case history with thoughtful and directed questioning is essential, as is an engaging approach with the patient. It is important to talk to the patient. Explaining procedures reduces the patients' anxiety levels, and allows participation in the treatment process. Involving the patient is a key step, as you rely on feedback to locate the exact centre of the trigger point.

How do I know it's a trigger point?

You are looking for:

- Stiffness in the affected / host muscle;
- Spot tenderness (exquisite pain);
- A palpable taut nodule or band;
- Presence of referred pain;
- Reproduction of the patients' symptoms (accurate).

What applicator should I use for palpation?

- Finger pads palpation: remember to cut your finger nails (shorter is better);
- Flat palpation: use the fingertips to slide around the patients' skin across muscle fibres;
- Pincer palpation: pinch the belly of the muscle between the thumb and the other fingers, rolling muscle fibres back and forth;
- Flat hand palpation: useful in the abdominal region (viscera);
- Elbow: allows stronger leverage which can be an advantage.

What equipment do I need?

- A *dermometer* to accurately measure reduced skin resistance (needs calibration);
- An *algometer* for measuring point tenderness and pain generated by pressure.

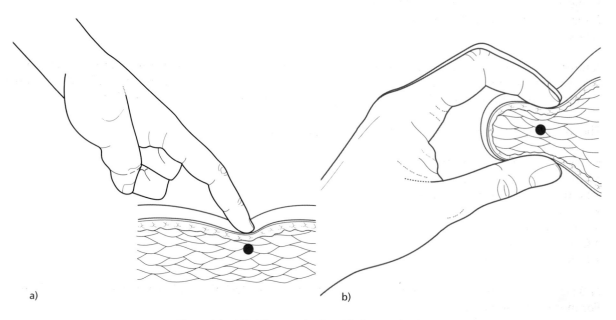

a)   b)

Figure 4.1: a) Flat finger palpation, b) pincer palpation.

The 'Jump and Twitch' Signs

This was first described in 1949 (Good, 1949; Kraft *et al.*, 1968). At first you should discover that it is easier to locate a *central* trigger point. Firmly pressing it produces *exquisite pain* and often causes the patient to *jump* away. The pain from an active *central* trigger point commonly causes a specific referred pain pattern. This is a distinct pattern away from the point of pressure. In the therapeutic context, this pattern often re-produces the pain felt by the patient.

Using a quick *snapping* pincer palpation or inserting a needle into a trigger point will often elicit a localized *twitch* response within the muscle.[25] This twitch may be due to the increased irritability of pain fibres as described above. You will find the patterns of referred pain in Chapters 5–10.

Injections vs Dry Needling

Dry needling is as effective as injection when it comes to relief of trigger point symptoms, but may leave a longer period of post injection soreness. The following table offers some ideas as to when to consider injection:

	Injection	Manual methods
Unexperienced therapist	Not recommended	Recommended
Invasive	Yes	No
Quick response to treatment	Yes	May require several sessions
Enables self-management	No	Yes
Point always accessible	No	Yes
Patient has low pain threshold	Yes	No
Patient is needle shy	No	Yes

Table 3: When to inject versus manual methods.

There are three different approaches to needling:[25]

1. Injection of a local anaesthetic (alone);
2. Injection with Botulinum toxin A;
3. Dry needling.

A number of injections may be required although sometimes one is sufficient. Small amounts (<1 ml) of a non-myotoxic anaesthetic are recommended. A local *twitch* response is a reliable indication of the correct position for needling. EMG monitoring allows increased accuracy and specificity.

The following have been suggested for use when injecting:

- Procaine hydrochloride 1% solution;
- Lidocaine hydrochloride (0.5%);
- Long-acting local anaesthetics;
- Isotonic saline;
- Epinephrin;
- Corticosteroid;
- Botulinum toxin A.

N.B.: It is not within the remit of this book to offer technical advice for such procedures. For more information, *see*[25].

Dry Needling Technique

In comparative studies, dry needling has been demonstrated to be as effective as injecting an anaesthetic solution (procaine hydrochloride or lidocaine hydrochloride) in de-activating trigger points. In these studies, however, dry needling caused localized soreness within 2–8 hours of injection. This soreness may be of a significantly greater intensity and / or duration than treatment with a wet injection.

- Locate trigger point and insert needle – watch for twitch response;
- Leave for up to 2 minutes, twiddling if necessary;
- Acupuncture needles may be used (8–15cm).

Spray and Stretch Technique

The technique of spray and stretch using ethyl chloride spray was first described by Hans Kraus (1952). Kraus used the technique for treating aches and sprains in wrestlers. Since then, techniques have been developed to treat almost all trigger points. These techniques are the *'single most effective non-invasive methods'* for de-activating trigger points.[25] Ethyl chloride spray is highly flammable, and toxic, and is considerably colder than is necessary. It is volatile and has accidentally killed several patients and doctors. Vapocoolents such as fluori-methane spray are a safer alternative, although being a fluorocarbon it may effect the ozone layer. The recommended product is *Gebauer's spray and stretch* as it is non-toxic and non-flammable.

The basic technique is quite straightforward as it does not require the same precise localization of trigger points as for an injection; instead you need only to locate and identify the affected / host muscle to release its fibres. However, it is advisable to locate the trigger point with palpation as this re-assures the patient as to the efficacy. There are two steps to this technique: 1. **Spray** – performed first; this is a distraction for the more important step of; 2. **Stretch** – is the therapeutic component of the technique.

1. Two to three sweeps of spray are applied to the affected / host muscle whilst extending the muscle gently to its full stretch length;

2. The spray is aimed out of the inverted bottle nozzle at 30° to the skin in a fine jet over a distance of about 30–50cm (do not aim at a single spot).

Situations when to use the spray and stretch technique include:

- Young children;
- Needle shy patient;
- Immediately after trigger point injection;
- Post-hemiplegic – stroke rehabilitation;
- Immediately following major trauma (e.g. fracture, dislocation);
- After whiplash injury;
- In a patient with myofascial trigger points and hyperuricaemia (excess uric acid);
- Chronic or inhibition resistant trigger points;
- Attachment trigger points;
- After sprains and burns.

Hints and Tips

- Locating the central trigger point which causes a precise referred pain pattern is recommended as it gives the patient a rationale to accept treatment;
- Make sure the patient has recently eaten, as hypoglycaemia aggravates trigger points;
- Have a warmish surgery / room;
- Use a blanket to cover the body and areas not being cooled, as muscle warmth is more conducive to muscle relaxation;
- Remember to cover the eyes where appropriate;
- DO NOT aim at a single spot as this can burn or cause urticaria;
- DO NOT force a stretch;
- If the patient is apprehensive, ask them to focus on their breathing;
- Test range of motion before and after the spray and stretch technique;
- Make sure that the muscle to be treated is fully relaxed and support it where possible; treatment can be performed sitting, side lying, prone or supine;
- To get a full stretch, you should anchor one side of the muscle, and move the other (passively).

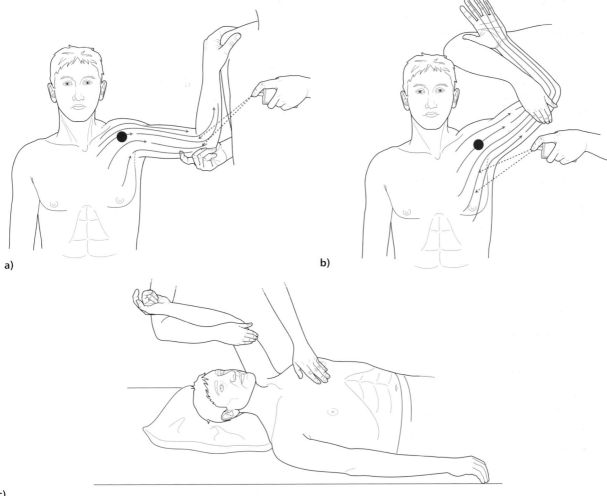

a)

b)

c)

Figure 4.2: Spray and stretch technique for pectoralis major.

Hands-on Therapy Trigger Point Release Protocols

Stretch and Release Techniques

These methods directly involve the patient, asking them to actively contract the affected / host muscle and then to relax it. This sequence forms the basis for several extremely effective inhibitory techniques:

- Post-isometric relaxation;
- Reciprocal inhibition;
- Contract and relax / hold and relax;
- Muscle energy / positional release.

These techniques are effective if you consider the concept of an over-stimulated motor end plate. Utilizing contraction and relaxation whilst fixing through the trigger point may well 'normalize' the sarcomere length. This sets in place a cascade, releasing the affected actin and myosin, and reducing the energy crisis. In this case, taking up the slack whilst inhibiting the trigger point (as in *positional release techniques*) may be particularly useful. Here, I will explore some of these techniques.

Post-isometric Relaxation (PIR) Technique

This technique was introduced by Karel Lewit (1981). The proposed complete technique incorporates the use of co-ordinated eye and respiratory movements (reflex augmentation).

- Identify the trigger point;
- Position the patient in a comfortable position where the affected / host muscle can undergo full excursion;
- Using 10–25% of their power ask the patient to contract the affected / host muscle at its maximal pain-free length, whilst applying isometric resistance for 3–10 seconds; stabilize the body part to prevent muscle shortening;
- Ask the patient to relax the muscle or 'let it go';
- During this relaxation phase, gently lengthen the muscle by taking-up the slack to the point of resistance (passive) – note any changes in length;
- Repeat several times (usually 3).

Reciprocal Inhibition Technique

This is an indirect technique relying on the agonist-antagonist neurological reflex. It is often used to augment other techniques, adding the 'finishing touch':

- The affected / host muscle is identified and taken into relaxation;
- The antagonist muscle is then contracted against 35–45% isometric resistance.

Contract and Relax / Hold and Relax Techniques

Originally taught by osteopaths Knott and Voss (1968), these techniques were devised to increase the passive range of motion of markedly stiff joints. The principles behind the techniques have a direct relevance to myofascial trigger point therapy, because as we have discussed, muscle tightness is often a sign of active or latent trigger points:

- Identify the trigger point;
- Position the patient in a comfortable position, where the affected / host muscle can undergo full excursion;
- Take the stiff joint to a comfortable near end-point, and ask the patient to actively contract the affected / host muscle;
- Gently resist this voluntary contraction;
- Allow relaxation;
- During this phase, passively stretch the joint to a new (increased) end point.

Modifications – Muscle Energy / Positional Release Techniques

These are osteopathic techniques which can be divided into three distinct approaches (Kuchera and Kuchera 1994). In all cases, first identify the trigger point:

1. Isometric Contraction Technique

- Hold or fix through the trigger point of the affected / host muscle;
- Ask the patient to actively contract the muscle without any resistance;
- Hold until a softening is palpated in the trigger point;
- Actively and passively stretch the muscle.

2. Isotonic Contraction Technique

- Hold or fix through the trigger point of the affected / host muscle;
- Ask the patient to actively contract the muscle at about 35–45%, whilst *you* resist / fix against it;
- Hold until a softening is palpated in the trigger point.

3. Isolytic Contraction Technique

- Hold or fix through the trigger point of the affected / host muscle;
- Ask the patient to actively contract the muscle at about 10–25%, whilst *you* resist it;
- Overcome this resistance, actively pushing against the muscle into eccentric contraction;
- Hold until a softening is palpated in the trigger point.

Massage Techniques

Inhibition-Ischaemic Compression Technique

This is the best technique to use on an active central trigger point. It involves locating the trigger point which causes a specific referred pain pattern (preferably reproducing the patients' symptoms) and applying a direct inhibitory pressure to the point. Although called ischaemic, it is now commonly accepted that you do not need to compress the trigger point to the point of ischaemia! This technique is effective, but is best used in conjunction with other stretch and release techniques. I have included a protocol which incorporates current approach.

I find it easier not to push or press on the trigger point, but to lean on it! This literally means to find the point, and lean weight through the applicator rather than push. This is much more comfortable for you and the patient.

- Identify and locate the trigger point;
- Position the patient in a comfortable position, where the affected / host muscle can undergo full excursion;
- Apply *gentle, gradual* increasing pressure to the trigger point whilst lengthening the affected / host muscle until you hit a palpable *barrier*;
- This should be experienced by the patient as discomfort and **NOT** pain;
- Apply sustained pressure until you feel the trigger point soften. This can take from seconds to minutes;
- Repeat, increasing the pressure on the trigger point until you meet the *next barrier*, and so on;
- To achieve a better result, you can try to change the direction of pressure during these repetitions.

   Tip! Don't come away too quickly as this can irritate the trigger point and make the symptoms worse. Feel, don't think!

Deep Stroking Massage Technique

Being more specific as it is more directed than the spray and stretch technique, it is also considered by most authorities to be the safest, and most effective hands-on method for treatment.[25]

- Position the patient in a comfortable position where the affected / host muscle can undergo full excursion;
- Lubricate the skin if required;
- Identify and locate the trigger point or taut band;
- Position your thumb / applicator just beyond the taut band, and re-enforce with your other hand;
- Apply gentle pressure to the trigger point whilst stroking in one direction only;
- This should be experienced by the patient as discomfort and **NOT** pain;
- Apply sustained pressure until you feel the trigger point soften, and continue stroking in the same direction towards the attachment of the taut band;
- Repeat this stroking in the opposite direction.

   Tip! Don't stroke too quickly or deeply as this can irritate the trigger point and rupture the sarcomere, making the symptoms worse.

A modification to the deep stroking massage technique is *strumming*, where the applicator is dragged perpendicularly across the taut band of muscle fibres. This is performed slowly and rhythmically using a light contact and pausing on the trigger point when it is palpated. It is especially useful for treating the *medial pterygoid* and the *masseter* muscles.

Frequently Asked Questions (FAQs)

What is the direction of force?

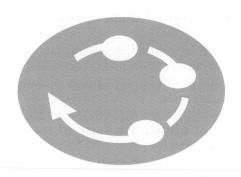

I have indicated the location of the main trigger points on the muscle diagrams in this book; these are for reference only and are not always accurate. It may be more helpful to think of the points as zones where you are most likely to find the trigger point. I have tried to represent this by the idea of a hot zone; the trigger point is located somewhere in this zone. You need to find the direction of pressure that where possible, reproduces the exact pain of which the patient is complaining. It often amazes me that a slight change in the direction of the pressure can cause a totally different pain elsewhere. Ask the patient to tell you when you are 'there.'

Figure 4.3: Hot zones.

How do I know when I've done enough?

Hold the trigger point until either the; a) patient's pain diminishes massively, or, b) trigger point softens or evaporates beneath your pressure.

Follow all deep work with a gentle generalized effleurage massage. The area where you did the deep work may still be tender but do not avoid it. This will help to dispel pain-inducing toxins from the area and stimulate the repair of the fascia.

How much pressure do I use?

This is something that comes with experience, but as a rule of thumb the more painful the tissue, the slower and deeper the pressure. In all cases, the key words are *'work slowly'* and *'thoroughly'*.

Another factor which determines the amount of force which you should apply is the muscle type (red / white fibre) and morphology of the patient. This will affect the depth of treatment. If the patient is 'stocky', I would expect to have to work quite vigorously. If they are slight, you won't need to use as much force to affect a change in the tissues.

Are the trigger points and referred pain patterns the same for everyone?

Generally yes, however the following will have an effect on the pattern:

- Ageing;
- Posture;
- Obesity;
- Anorexia;
- Scar tissue;
- Myofascial strain patterns;
- Congenital anomaly;
- Type of muscle fibre;
- Direction / orientation of muscle fibre;
- Type of muscle morphology (fusiform, etc.);
- Chronicity of trigger point.

What effect does obesity, anorexia, and scar tissue have?

These factors will change the fat / muscle ratio and skew the position of the trigger points. They will also have an effect on the planes of the fascia, and hence the location of the trigger points. Similarly, scar tissue or keloid may cause a deviation in the myofascial strain pattern and hence the location of the trigger point.

What about the type of muscle fibre, or the orientation of muscle fibre?

Depending on where they are in the body and the job they have to do, muscle fibres are arranged into various structures (*see* page 26). This allows the muscles to generate either more force, or a more specific force. Locating a central trigger point will therefore vary according to the arrangement of muscle fibres within any given muscle. In the multipennate fibre arrangement, for example, several trigger points may exist in the middle of each of the functional components.

Will bruising occur?

Bruising may occur if the patient is on blood thinning medication. With time and experience, bruising becomes increasingly rare. In my experience, it is not the depth (force) of treatment that will cause the skin to bruise; but that it is done too quickly (velocity).

> **Tip!** Try to feel the muscles and tender nodules beneath the skin and build up the pressure slowly; do not come away too quickly. Arnica creams and tablets may reduce the incidence and severity of bruising.

What creams or lotions can I use?

In general, it is better to avoid oils as they may cause you to slide off from the pressure points once you have found them. I use plain blue *Nivea*™ cream. Alternatively, Arnica cream or plain aqueous cream mixed with some vitamin E oil may be sufficient. Also petroleum gel or massage oil may be used, if the patient has a lanolin allergy.

What is the frequency of treatment?

In my experience, for hands-on therapy you should perform three treatment sessions one week apart; another session four weeks later, and a final session twelve weeks after this. This is in line with the mechanical repair of fascia. You may want to review the patient again after this. Injections and dry needling have a much quicker action.[25]

5

Muscles of the Scalp, Face and Neck

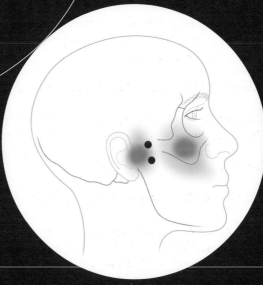

EPICRANIUS (OCCIPITOFRONTALIS)

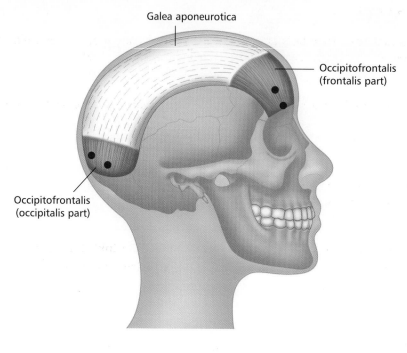

Galea aponeurotica

Occipitofrontalis
(frontalis part)

Occipitofrontalis
(occipitalis part)

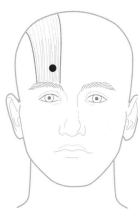

Frontalis part

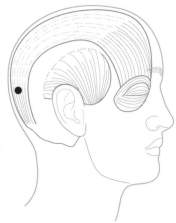

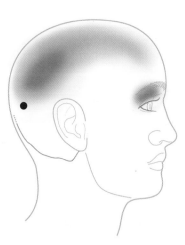

Occipitalis part

Greek, *epi-*, upon; **Latin**, *cranium*, skull.

This muscle is effectively two muscles (occipitalis and frontalis), united by an aponeurosis called the *galea aponeurotica*, so named because it forms what resembles a helmet upon the skull.

Origin
Occipitalis: lateral two-thirds of superior nuchal line of occipital bone. Mastoid process of temporal bone.
Frontalis: galea aponeurotica.

Insertion
Occipitalis: galea aponeurotica (a sheet-like tendon leading to frontal belly).
Frontalis: fascia and skin above eyes and nose.

Action
Occipitalis: pulls scalp backward. Assists frontal belly to raise eyebrows and wrinkle forehead.
Frontalis: pulls scalp forwards. Raises eyebrows and wrinkles skin of forehead horizontally.

Nerve
Facial **V11** nerve.

Basic functional movement
Example: Raises eyebrows (wrinkles skin of forehead horizontally).

Indications
Headache. Pain (back of head). Cannot sleep on back / pillow. Earache. Pain behind eye, eyebrow, and eyelid. Visual activity.

Referred pain patterns
Occipitalis: pain in the lateral and anterior scalp; diffuse into back of head and into orbit.
Frontalis: localized pain with some referral upwards and over forehead on the same side.

Differential diagnosis
Scalp tingling. Greater occipital nerve entrapment.

Also consider
Suboccipital muscles. Clavicular division of sternocleidomastoideus. Semispinalis capitis.

Advice to patient
Avoid frowning and wrinkling of forehead.

Techniques

Spray and stretch			
Injections	✓		

Dry needling	✓		
Trigger point release	✓	✓	

ORBICULARIS OCULI

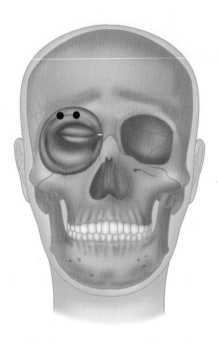

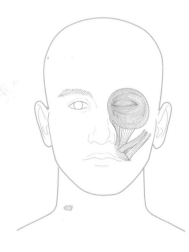

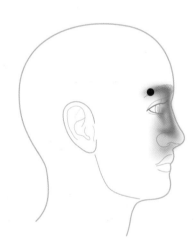

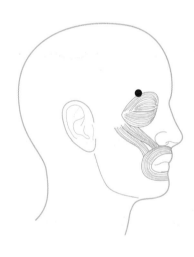

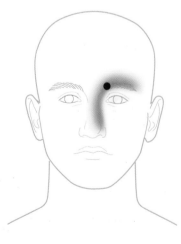

Latin, *orbis*, orb, circle; *oculi*, of the eye.

This complex and extremely important muscle consists of three parts, which together form an important protective mechanism surrounding the eye.

Orbital part

Origin
Frontal bone. Medial wall of orbit (on maxilla).

Insertion
Circular path around orbit, returning to origin.

Action
Strongly closes eyelids (firmly 'screws up' the eye).

Nerve
Facial **V11** nerve (temporal and zygomatic branches).

Palpebral part (in eyelids)

Latin, pertaining to an eyelid.

Origin
Medial palpebral ligament.

Insertion
Lateral palpebral ligament into zygomatic bone.

Action
Gently closes eyelids (and comes into action involuntarily, as in blinking).

Nerve
Facial **V11** nerve (temporal and zygomatic branches).

Lacrimal part (behind medial palpebral ligament and lacrimal sac)

Latin, pertaining to the tears.

Origin
Lacrimal bone.

Insertion
Lateral palpebral raphe.

Action
Dilates lacrimal sac and brings lacrimal canals onto surface of eye.

Nerve
Facial **V11** nerve (temporal and zygomatic branches).

Indications
Headache. Migraine. Trigeminal neuralgia. Eyestrain. 'Twitching' eyes. Poor eyesight. Drooping eyelid. Sinus pain.

Referred pain patterns
Palpebral: localized 'searing' pain above eye and up to ipsilateral nostril.
Lacrimal: into eye, sinus pain, bridge of nose pain. Ice cream often reproduces eye pain / headache.

Differential diagnosis
Ptosis – Horner's syndrome.

Also consider
Digastric. Temporalis. Trapezius. Spleneii, and post cervical muscles. Often associated with sternocleidomastoideus.

Advice to patient
Check eyesight regularly. Increase sleep / rest. Regular breaks when driving or looking at VDU screen. Are glasses too tight on bridge of nose?

Techniques

Spray and stretch	☐ ☐	Dry needling ✓ ✓
Injections ✓ ✓		Trigger point release ✓ ✓

MASSETER

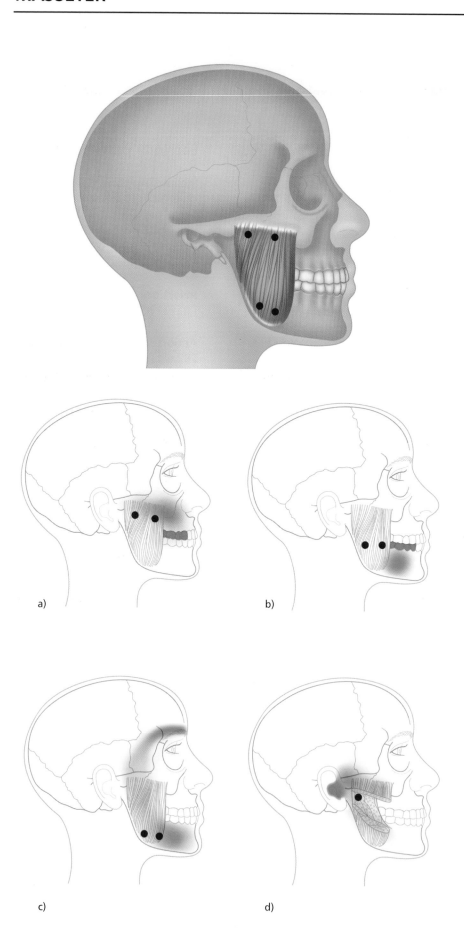

a)

b)

c)

d)

Greek, *maseter*, chewer.

The masseter is the most superficial muscle of mastication, easily felt when the jaw is clenched.

Origin
Zygomatic process of maxilla. Medial and inferior surfaces of zygomatic arch.

Insertion
Angle of ramus of mandible. Coronoid process of mandible.

Action
Closes jaw. Clenches teeth. Assists in side to side movement of mandible.

Nerve
Trigeminal **V** nerve (mandibular division).

Basic functional movement
Chewing food.

Indications
Trismus (severely restricted jaw). TMJ pain. Tension / stress headache. Ear pain. Ipsilateral tinnitus. Dental pain.

Referred pain patterns
Superficial: eyebrow, maxilla and mandible (anterior). Upper and lower molar teeth.
Deep: ear and TMJ.

Differential diagnosis
TMJ pain / syndrome. Tinnitus. Trismus.

Also consider
Ipsilateral temporalis. Medial pterygoid. Contralateral masseter. Sternocleidomastoideus.

Advice to patients
Stop tooth grinding (bite plates). Work posture (telephone). Posture of head-neck-tongue. Stop chewing gum / ice / nails.

Techniques

Spray and stretch	✓	Dry needling	✓
Injections	✓ ✓	Trigger point release	✓ ✓

N.B. vapours in asthmatics

TEMPORALIS

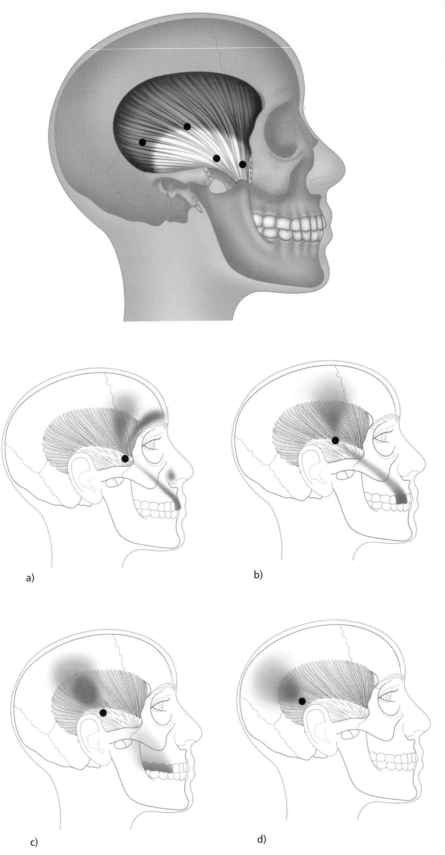

a)

b)

c)

d)

Self stretch

Latin, pertaining to the lateral side of the head, time.

Origin
Temporal fossa, including parietal, temporal and frontal bones. Temporal fascia.

Insertion
Coronoid process of mandible. Anterior border of ramus of mandible.

Action
Closes jaw. Clenches teeth. Assists in side to side movement of mandible.

Nerve
Anterior and posterior deep temporal nerves from the trigeminal **V** nerve (mandibular division).

Basic functional movement
Chewing food.

Indications
Headache. Toothache. TMJ syndrome. Hypersensitivity of teeth. Prolonged dental work. Eyebrow pain.

Referred pain patterns
Upper incisors and supraorbital ridge. Maxillary teeth and mid temple pain. TMJ and mid temple pain. Localized (backwards and upwards).

Differential diagnosis
Temporalis tendonitis. Polymyalgia rheumatica. Temporal arteritis (GCA).

Also consider
Upper trapezius. Sternocleidomastoideus. Masseter.

Advice to patients
Gum chewing or hard substance chewing. Tongue position. Air conditioning in car / at work. Correcting of the head – forward posture. Stretch.

Techniques

Spray and stretch	✓	✓	Dry needling	✓	
Injections	✓	✓	Trigger point release	✓	✓

PTERYGOIDEUS LATERALIS (Lateral Pterygoid)

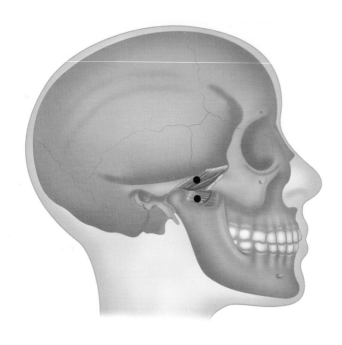

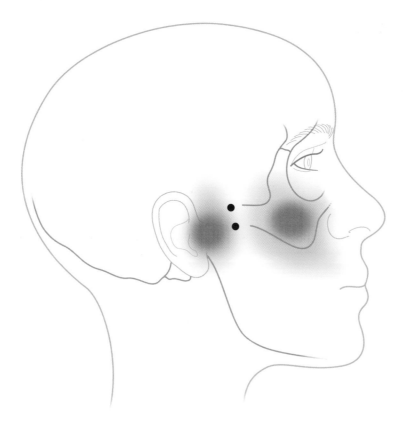

Greek, *pterygodes*, like a wing; **Latin**, *lateral*, to the side.

The superior head of this muscle is sometimes called *sphenomeniscus*, because it inserts into the disc of the temporomandibular joint.

Origin
Superior head: lateral surface of greater wing of sphenoid.
Inferior head: lateral surface of lateral pterygoid plate of sphenoid.

Insertion
Superior head: capsule and articular disc of the temporomandibular joint.
Inferior head: neck of mandible.

Action
Protrudes mandible. Opens mouth. Moves mandible from side to side (as in chewing).

Nerve
Trigeminal **V** nerve (mandibular division).

Basic functional movement
Chewing food.

Indications
TMJ syndrome. Cranio-mandibular pain. Problems chewing / masticating. Tinnitus. Sinusitis. Decreased jaw opening.

Referred pain patterns
Two zones of pain; 1) TMJ in a 1cm localized zone; 2) zygomatic arch in a 3–4cm zone.

Differential diagnosis
Arthritic TMJ. Anatomical variations of TMJ. Tic douloureux *(*trigeminal neuralgia). Shingles.

Also consider
TMJ. Atlanto-occipital joint facets. Neck muscles. Masseter. Medial pterygoid. Temporalis (anterior).

Advice to patient
Chew on both sides of mouth. Avoid gum chewing / nail biting. Bite-guard, phone-in-neck postures.

Techniques

Spray and stretch	✓		Dry needling		
Injections	✓	✓	Trigger point release	✓	✓

PTERYGOIDEUS MEDIALIS (Medial Pterygoid)

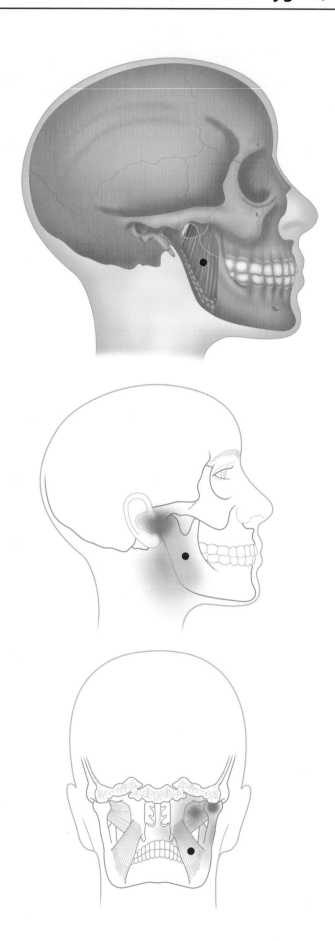

PTERYGOIDEUS MEDIALIS (Medial Pterygoid)

Greek, *pterygodes*, like a wing; **Latin**, *medius*, middle.

This muscle mirrors the masseter muscle in both its position and action, with the ramus of the mandible positioned between the two muscles.

Origin
Medial surface of lateral pterygoid plate of the sphenoid bone. Pyramidal process of the palatine bone. Tuberosity of maxilla.

Insertion
Medial surface of the ramus and the angle of the mandible.

Action
Elevates and protrudes the mandible. Therefore it closes the jaw and assists in side to side movement of the mandible, as in chewing.

Nerve
Trigeminal **V** nerve (mandibular division).

Basic functional movement
Chewing food.

Indications
Throat pain. Odynophagia. TMJ syndrome. Lock jaw. Inability to fully open jaw. ENT pain. Excessive dental treatment.

Referred pain patterns
Pain in throat, mouth, and pharynx. Localized zone about TMJ radiating broadly down ramus of jaw towards the clavicle.

Differential diagnosis
TMJ syndrome. ENT pathologies. GI referral, e.g. Barrett's syndrome (oesophagus). Bruxism.

Also consider
Masseter. Temporalis. Lateral pterygoid. Tongue. Sternocleidomastoideus. Digastric. Longus capitis. Longus colli. Platysma. Clavipectoral fascia.

Advice to patient
Head postures. Chew on both sides of mouth. Bite guard (soft). Avoid chewing gum / nails.

Techniques

Spray and stretch	✓		Dry needling		
Injections	✓	✓	Trigger point release (internal and external)	✓	✓

DIGASTRICUS

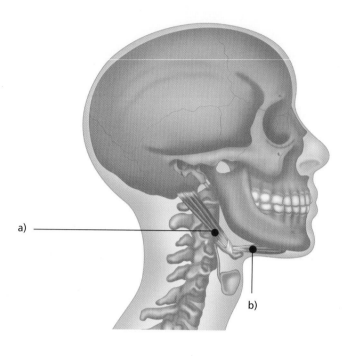

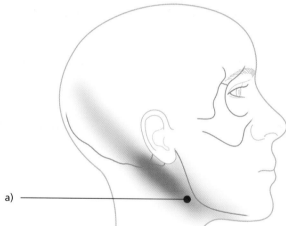

Posterior trigger point

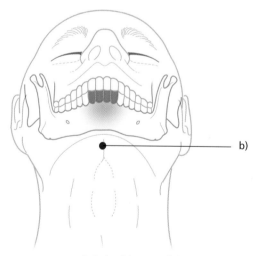

Anterior trigger point

Latin, having two bellies.

Origin
Anterior belly: digastric fossa on inner side of lower border of mandible, near symphysis.
Posterior belly: mastoid notch of temporal bone.

Insertion
Body of hyoid bone via a fascial sling over an intermediate tendon.

Action
Raises hyoid bone. Depresses and retracts mandible as in opening the mouth.

Nerve
Anterior belly: mylohyoid nerve, from trigeminal **V** nerve (mandibular division).
Posterior belly: facial (**V11**) nerve.

Indications
Throat pain. Dental pain (four lower incisors). Headache. Jaw pain. Renal tubular acidosis. Prolonged / extensive dental work (blurred vision and dizziness). Lower mouth opening.

Referred pain patterns
Anterior: lower four incisor teeth, tongue, and lip, occasionally to chin.
Posterior: strong 2cm zone around mastoid and vaguely zone to chin and throat, occasionally to scalp.

Differential diagnosis
Dental problems – malocclusion. Hyoid bone. Thyroid problems. Thymus gland. Sinusitis. Carotid artery.

Also consider
Sternocleidomastoideus. Sternothyroid. Mylohyoid. Stylohyoid. Longus colli. Longus capitis. Geniohyoid. Cervical vertebrae. Temporalis. Masseter.

Advice to patient
Breathing patterns. Bruxism. Head postures.

Techniques

Spray and stretch	✓		Dry needling		
Injections	✓	✓	Trigger point release	✓	✓

SCALENUS ANTERIOR, MEDIUS, POSTERIOR

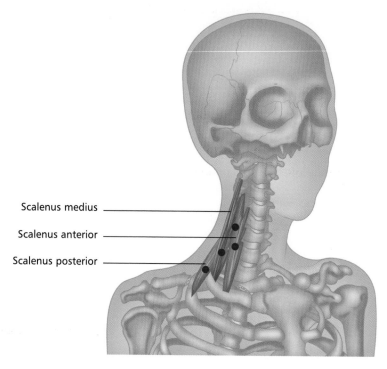

Scalenus medius

Scalenus anterior

Scalenus posterior

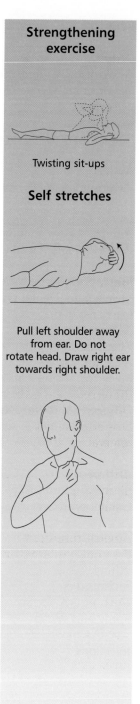

Strengthening exercise

Twisting sit-ups

Self stretches

Pull left shoulder away from ear. Do not rotate head. Draw right ear towards right shoulder.

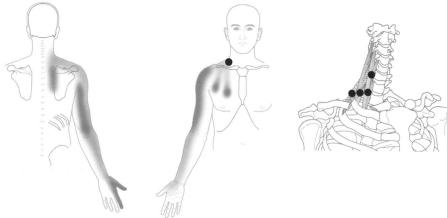

Scalenus medius, anterior, posterior and referred pain patterns

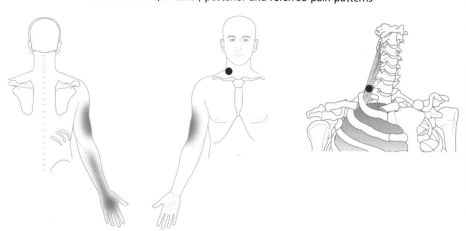

Scalenus medius and referred pain patterns

Greek, *skalenos*, uneven; **Latin**, *anterior*, before; *medius*, middle; *posterior*, behind.

Origin
Transverse processes of cervical vertebrae.

Insertion
Anterior and medius: first rib.
Posterior: second rib.

Action
Acting together: flex neck. Raise first rib during a strong inhalation.
Individually: laterally flex and rotate neck.

Nerve
Ventral rami of cervical nerves, C3–C8.

Basic functional movement
Primarily muscles of inspiration.

Indications
Back, shoulder and arm pain. Thoracic outlet syndrome. Scalene syndrome. Oedema in the hand. Phantom limb pain. Asthma, chronic lung disease. Whiplash. 'Restless neck'. Irritability.

Referred pain patterns
Anterior: persistent aching, pectoralis region to the nipple.
Posterior: upper medial border of scapula.
Lateral: front and back of the arm to the thumb and index finger.

Differential diagnosis
Brachial plexus. Subclavian vessels. Cervical discs (C5–C6). Thoracic outlet syndrome. Angina. Carpal tunnel syndrome. Upper trapezius. Sternocleidomastoideus. Splenius capitis.

Advice to patient
Use of pillows. Swimming. Backpacks. Heavy breasts. Warm scarfs. Warmth. Moist heat. Pulling and lifting.

Techniques

Spray and stretch	✓	✓	Dry needling		
Injections	✓	✓	Trigger point release	✓	

STERNOCLEIDOMASTOIDEUS

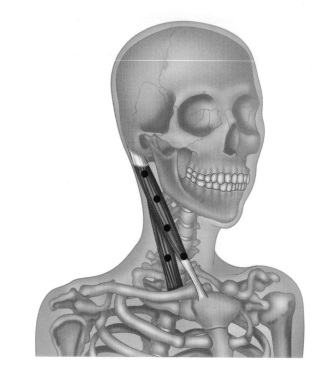

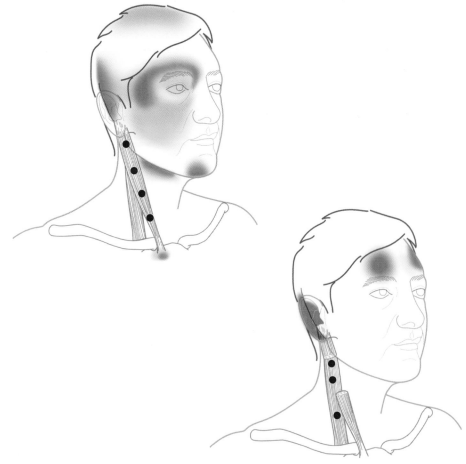

Strengthening exercise

Sit-ups

Self stretch

Turn head to right.
Repeat on opposite side.

Greek, *sternon*, sternum; *kleidos*, key, clavicle; *mastoid*, breast-shaped, mastoid process.

This muscle is a long strap muscle with two heads. It is sometimes injured at birth, and may be partly replaced by fibrous tissue that contracts to produce a torticollis (wry neck).

Origin
Sternal head: anterior surface of manubrium of sternum.
Clavicular head: upper surface of medial third of clavicle.

Insertion
Outer surface of mastoid process of temporal bone. Lateral third of superior nuchal line of occipital bone.

Action
Contraction of both sides together: flexes neck and draws head forward, as in raising the head from a pillow. Raises sternum, and consequently the ribs, superiorly during deep inhalation.
Contraction of one side: tilts the head towards the same side. Rotates head to face the opposite side, (and also upwards as it does so).

Nerve
Accessory **X1** nerve; with sensory supply for proprioception from cervical nerves C2 and C3.

Basic functional movement
Examples: Turning head to look over your shoulder. Raising head from pillow.

Indications
Tension headache. Whiplash. Stiff neck. Atypical facial neuralgia. Hangover headache. Postural dizziness. Altered (hemifacial sympathetics). Lowered spatial awareness. Ptosis.

Referred pain patterns
Sternal: pain in occiput radiating anteriorly to eyebrow, cheek, and throat (eye and sinus).
Clavicular: frontal headache, earache, mastoid pain (dizziness and spatial awareness).

Differential diagnosis
Trigeminal neuralgia. Facial neuralgia. Vestibulocochlear problems. Lymphadenopathy. Levator scapulae. Upper trapezius. Splenius capitis.

Advice to patient
Breathing efficacy. Number of pillows. Work posture. Head posture. TV posture.

Techniques

Spray and stretch	✓	✓	Dry needling*	✓	
Injections*	✓		Trigger point release	✓	✓

* vascular considerations

6

Muscles of the Trunk and Spine

ERECTOR SPINAE (SACROSPINALIS)

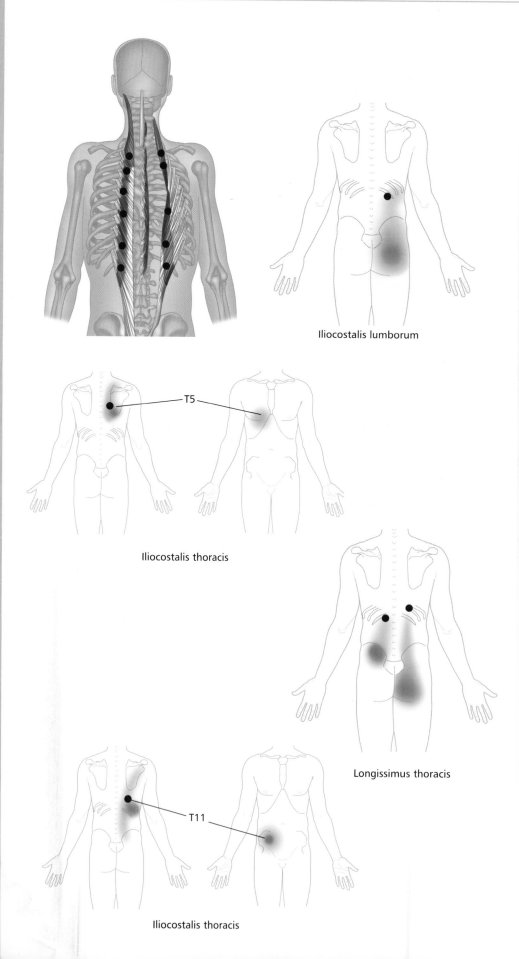

Iliocostalis lumborum

Iliocostalis thoracis

T5

Longissimus thoracis

T11

Iliocostalis thoracis

Strengthening exercises

Back extension (back raise)

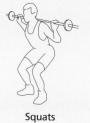

Lat. pull downs

Squats

Self stretches

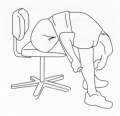

Move towel up back with each set of stretching.

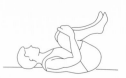

Pull knees into your chest and up towards your shoulders.

Latin, *sacrum*, sacred; *spinalis*, spinal.

The erector spinae, also called *sacrospinalis*, comprises three sets of muscles organised in parallel columns. From lateral to medial, they are: iliocostalis, longissimus and spinalis.

Origin
Slips of muscle arising from the sacrum. Iliac crest. Spinous and transverse processes of vertebrae. Ribs.

Insertion
Ribs. Transverse and spinous processes of vertebrae. Occipital bone.

Action
Extends and laterally flexes vertebral column (i.e. bending backwards and sideways).
Helps maintain correct curvature of spine in the erect and sitting positions. Steadies the vertebral column on the pelvis during walking.

Nerve
Dorsal rami of cervical, thoracic, and lumbar spinal nerves.

Basic functional movement
Keeps back straight (with correct curvatures). Therefore maintains posture.

Indications
Low back pain, especially after lifting. Reduced range of motion in the spine. Low back pain, either from sitting, standing or climbing stairs. Low grade back ache worsening towards the end of the day.

Referred pain patterns
Thoracic spine – iliocostalis: medially towards the spine, and anteriorly towards the abdomen.
Lumbar spine – iliocostalis: mid buttock.
Thoracic spine – iliocostalis: buttock and sacroiliac area.

Differential diagnosis
Angina. Visceral pain. Radiculopathy. Ligamentous, discogenic, sacroiliac. Piriformis.
Pathological: aortic aneurysm. Visceral pathology. Space occupying lesion. Pelvic inflammatory disease.

Advice to patient
Avoid 'sudden overload' when lifting. Do not lift when fatigued. Posture. Heat / hot baths.

Techniques

Spray and stretch	✓	✓	Dry needling	✓	✓
Injections	✓	✓	Trigger point release	✓	✓

POSTERIOR CERVICAL MUSCLES

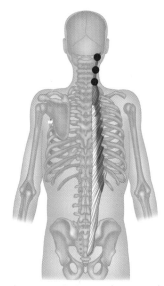

Longissimus capitis

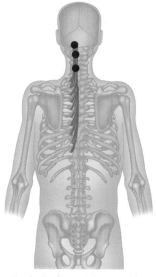

Semispinalis capitis / cervicis

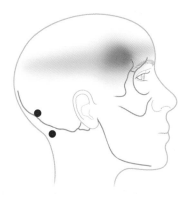

Semispinalis capitis (upper)

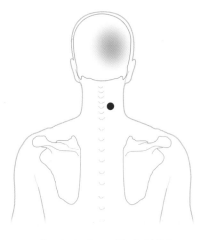

Semispinalis capitis (middle)

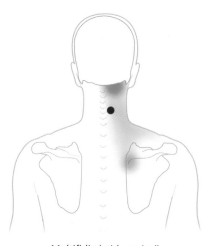

Multifidis (mid cervical)
Even though not mentioned here
(*see* also page 86), this muscle runs up
the spine as part of the erector spinae,
and so is relevant as part of the
posterior cervical muscles.

Strengthening exercise

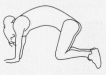

Back extension (back raise)

Self stretches

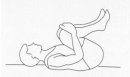

Arch your back as if being
drawn up by a piece
of string.

Pull knees into your chest
and up towards your
shoulders.

Latin, *longissimus*, longest; *capitis*, of the head; *semispinalis*, half spinal; *cervix*, neck.

Comprising longissimus capitis, semispinalis capitis, and semispinalis cervicis.

Origin
Longissimus capitis: transverse processes of upper five thoracic vertebrae, (T1–T5). Articular processes of lower three cervical vertebrae, (C5–C7).
Semispinalis cervicis: transverse processes of upper five or six thoracic vertebrae, (T1–T6).
Semispinalis capitis: transverse processes of lower four cervical and upper six or seven thoracic vertebrae, (C4–T7).

Insertion
Longissimus capitis: posterior part of mastoid process of temporal bone.
Semispinalis cervicis: spinous processes second to fifth cervical vertebrae, (C2–C5).
Semispinalis capitis: between superior and inferior nuchal lines of occipital bone.

Action
Longissimus capitis: extends and rotates head. Helps maintain correct curvature of thoracic and cervical spine in the erect and sitting positions.
Semispinalis cervicis: extends thoracic and cervical parts of vertebral column. Assists rotation of thoracic and cervical vertebrae.
Semispinalis capitis: most powerful extensor of the head. Assists in rotation of head.

Nerve
Longissimus capitis: dorsal rami of middle and lower cervical nerves.
Semispinalis cervicis: dorsal rami of thoracic and cervical nerves.
Semispinalis capitis: dorsal rami of cervical nerves.

Basic functional movement
Longissimus capitis: keeps upper back straight (with correct curvatures).
Semispinalis cervicis and capitis. Example: Looking up, or turning the head to look behind.

Indications
Headache. Neck pain and stiffness. Decreased cervical flexion. Suboccipital pain. Restricted neck rotation, often related to prolonged occupational positions. Whiplash. Pain on sleeping on certain pillows. 'Burning' in scalp.

Referred pain patterns
Several areas along the fibres, all radiating superiorly into head, skull and towards the frontal region.

Differential diagnosis
Cervical mechanical dysfunction. Spondyloarthropathy of facets. Vertebral artery syndrome. Discopathy (cervical) first rib dysfunction. Polymyalgia rheumatica. Rheumatoid arthritis. Osteoarthritis. Ankylosing spondylitis (seronegative spondyloarthropathy). Paget's disease. Psoriatic arthropathy.

Also consider
Trapezius. Erector spinae. Temporalis. Digastric. Infraspinatus. Levator scapulae. Sternocleidomastoideus. Splenius capitis. Splenius cervicis. Suboccipital muscles. Occipitalis.

Advice to patient
Occupational ergonomics. Posture. Eyewear. Use of ergonomic pillows. Heat and stretch. Explore bedding / pillows.

Techniques

Spray and stretch	✓ ✓	Dry needling	☐ ☐
Injections	✓ ☐	Trigger point release	✓ ☐

MULTIFIDIS / ROTATORES

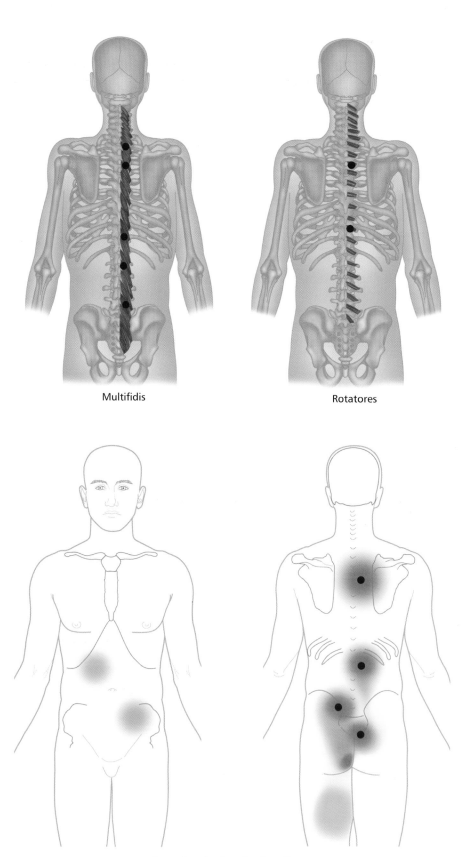

Multifidis

Rotatores

Examples of referred pain patterns.
Note the characteristic midline zones.

Latin, *multi*, many, much; *findere*, to split; *rot*, wheel.

Multifidis is the part of the transversospinalis group that lies in the furrow between the spines of the vertebrae and their transverse processes. It lies deep to semispinalis and erector spinae. Rotatores are the deepest layer of the transverspinalis group.

Origin

Multifidis: posterior surface of sacrum, between the sacral foramina and posterior superior iliac spine. Mamillary processes (posterior borders of superior articular processes) of all lumbar vertebrae. Transverse processes of all thoracic vertebrae. Articular processes of lower four cervical vertebrae.
Rotatores: transverse process of each vertebra.

Insertion

Multifidis: parts insert into spinous process two to four vertebrae superior to origin; overall including spinous processes of all the vertebrae from the fifth lumbar up to the axis, (L5–C2).
Rotatores: base of spinous process of adjoining vertebra above.

Action

Multifidis: protects vertebral joints from movements produced by the more powerful superficial prime movers. Extension, lateral flexion and rotation of vertebral column.
Rotatores: rotate and assist in extension of vertebral column.

Nerve

Dorsal rami of spinal nerves.

Basic functional movement

Helps maintain good posture and spinal stability during standing, sitting and all movements.

Indications

Deep / persistant low backache. Vertebral alignment problems. Facilitated segment – localized paraspinal erythema. Coccydynia.

Referred pain patterns

Multifidis: localized and anteriorly to abdomen. S1 leads to coccydynia.
Rotatores: localized to medial pain.

Differential diagnosis

Angina. Visceral pain. Radiculopathy. Ligamentous, discogenic, sacroiliac. Piriformis.
Pathological: aortic aneurysm. Visceral pathology. Space occupying lesion. Pelvic inflammatory disease.

Advice to patient

Posture. Kyphosis from working position. Number and type of pillows. Occupational considerations.

Techniques

Spray and stretch	✓ ✓	Dry needling ✓ ✓
Injections	✓ ✓	Trigger point release ✓ ✓

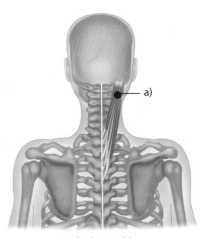

Splenius capitis

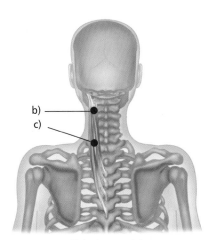

Splenius cervicis

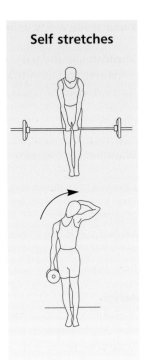

Self stretches

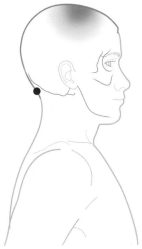

a) Splenius capitis

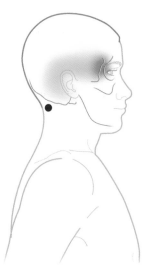

b) Splenius cervicis (upper)

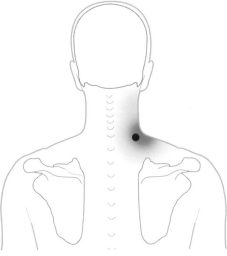

c) Splenius cervicis (lower)

Greek, *splenion*, bandage; **Latin**, *capitis*, of the head; *cervix*, neck.

Origin
Splenius capitis: lower part of ligamentum nuchae. Spinous processes of the seventh cervical vertebra, (C7 and upper three or four thoracic vertebrae, (T1–T4).
Splenius cervicis: spinous processes of the third to sixth thoracic vertebrae, (T3–T6).

Insertion
Splenius capitis: posterior aspect of mastoid process of temporal bone. Lateral part of superior nuchal line, deep to the attachment of the sternocleidomastoideus.
Splenius cervicis: posterior tubercles of transverse processes of the upper two or three cervical vertebrae, (C1–C3).

Action
Acting together: extend the head and neck.
Individually: laterally flexes neck. Rotates the face to the same side as contracting muscle.

Nerve
Dorsal rami of middle and lower cervical nerves.

Basic functional movement
Example: Looking up, or turning the head to look behind.

Indications
Headache. Neck pain. Eye pain. Blurred vision (rare). Whiplash. Pain from draught. Postural neck pain (occupational). 'Internal' skull pain. Neck stiffness. Decreased ipsilateral rotation.

Referred pain patterns
Splenius capitis: 3–5cm zone of pain in the centre of the vertex of the skull.
Splenius cervicis: a) upper: occipital diffuse pain radiating via the temporal region toward the ipsilateral eye; b) lower: ipsilateral pain in the nape of the neck.

Differential diagnosis
Other types of headache. First rib dysfunction. Torticollis. Optical problems (eyestrain). Neurological. Stress.

Also consider
Trapezius. Sternocleidomastoideus. Masseter. Temporalis. Multifidis. Semispinalis capitis. Suboccipital muscles. Occipitofrontalis. Levator scapulae.

Advice to patient
Avoid postural / maintaining factors, answering the telephone. Work posture. Self stretch programme. Glasses (type, try trifocals).

Techniques

Spray and stretch	✓ ✓	Dry needling	✓
Injections	✓	Trigger point release	✓ ✓

EXTERNAL OBLIQUE

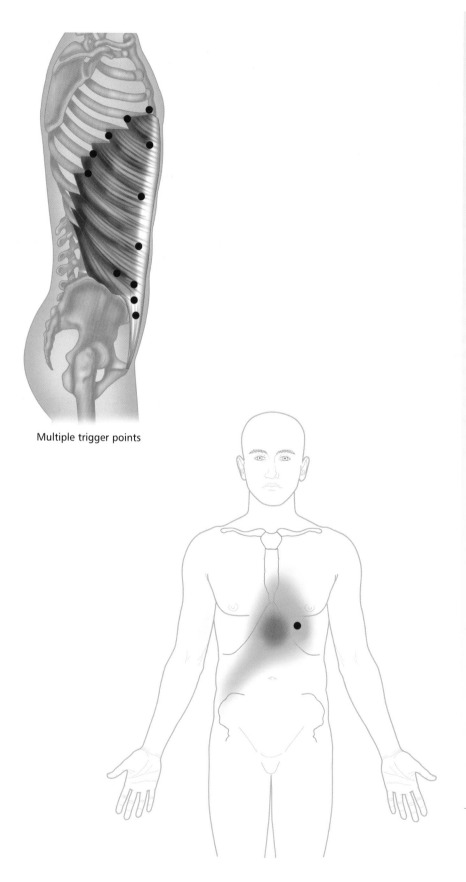

Multiple trigger points

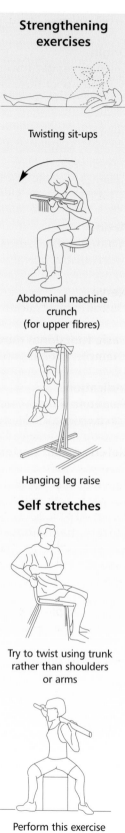

Strengthening exercises

Twisting sit-ups

Abdominal machine crunch (for upper fibres)

Hanging leg raise

Self stretches

Try to twist using trunk rather than shoulders or arms

Perform this exercise slowly, thus avoiding the tendency to use momentum

Latin, *obliquu*s, inclined, slanting; *externus*, external.

The posterior fibres of the external oblique are usually overlapped by the latissimus dorsi, but in some cases there is a space between the two, known as the *lumbar triangle*, situated just above the iliac crest. The lumbar triangle is a weak point in the abdominal wall.

Origin
Lower eight ribs.

Insertion
Anterior half of iliac crest, and into an abdominal aponeurosis that terminates in the linea alba (a tendinous band extending downwards from the sternum).

Action
Compresses abdomen, helping to support the abdominal viscera against the pull of gravity. Contraction of one side alone bends the trunk laterally to that side and rotates it to the opposite side.

Nerve
Ventral rami of thoracic nerves, T5–T12.

Basic functional movement
Example: Digging with a shovel.

Indications
Abdominal pain and tenderness. Groin pain. Testicular pain. Bladder pain. Nausea. Colic. Dysmenorrhoea. Diarrhoea. Viscerosomatic. Irritable bowel syndrome.

Referred pain patterns
Viscerosomatic.
Costal margin: abdominal pain to chest.
Lower lateral: testicular pain. Local pain.
Pubic rim: bladder pain. Frequency / retention (urine). Groin.

Differential diagnosis
Visceral pathology including; renal, hepatic, pancreatic, diverticular disease, colitis, appendicitis, hiatus hernia, peritoneal disease – pelvic inflammatory disease, ovarian, bladder.

Advice to patient
Occupational. Sports. Diet. Breathing. Pelvic floor, and core stability exercises.

Techniques

| Spray and stretch | ✓ | ✓ | Dry needling | ✓ | |
| Injections | ✓ | | Trigger point release | ✓ | ✓ |

TRANSVERSUS ABDOMINIS

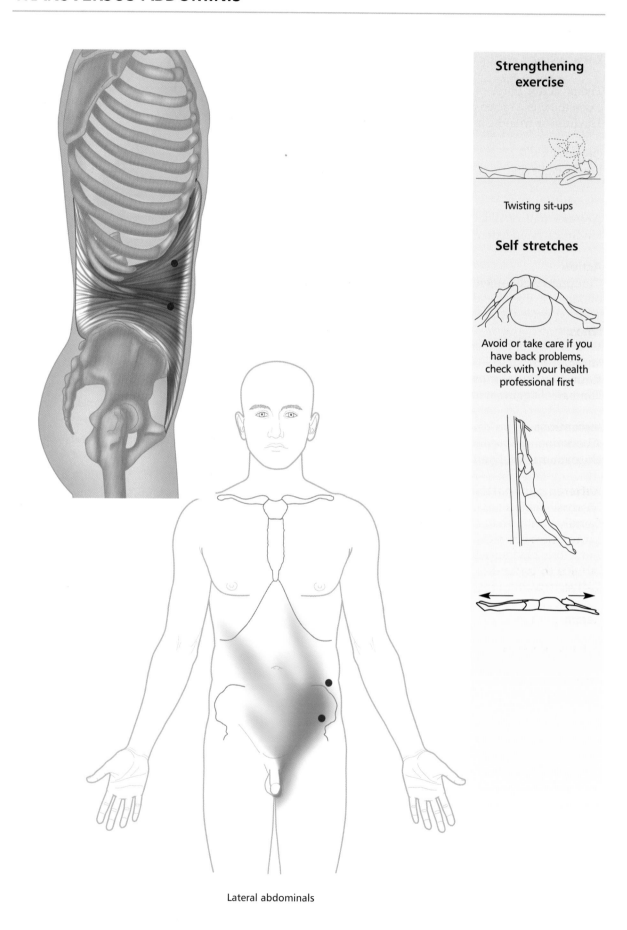

Strengthening exercise

Twisting sit-ups

Self stretches

Avoid or take care if you
have back problems,
check with your health
professional first

Lateral abdominals

Latin, *transversus*, across, crosswise; *abdominis*, belly / stomach.

Origin
Anterior two thirds of iliac crest. Lateral third of inguinal ligament. Thoracolumbar fascia. Costal cartilages of lower six ribs. Fascia covering iliopsoas.

Insertion
Xiphoid process and linea alba via an abdominal aponeurosis, the lower fibres of which ultimately attach to the pubic crest and pecten pubis via the conjoint tendon.

Action
Compresses abdomen, helping to support the abdominal viscera against the pull of gravity.

Nerve
Ventral rami of thoracic nerves, T7–T12, ilioinguinal and iliohypogastric nerves.

Basic functional movement
Important during forced expiration, sneezing and coughing. Helps maintain good posture.

Indications
Groin pain. Testicular pain. Heartburn. Nausea. Vomiting. Bloating. Diarrhoea. Discogenic pain from the lumbar spine.

Referred pain patterns
Costal margin: local quadrant pain often radiating into anterior abdomen.
Suprapubic: local pain often radiating medially and inferiorly to testes.

Differential diagnosis
Visceral pathology including; renal, hepatic, pancreatic, diverticular disease, colitis, appendicitis, hiatus hernia, peritoneal disease – pelvic inflammatory disease, ovarian, bladder, testicular pathology, e.g. varicocele, non-specific urethritis.

Advice to patient
Self stretch and strengthen to stabilise lumbar spine and support vascular activities. Posture and tone.

Techniques

Spray and stretch	✓		Dry needling	✓
Injections	✓		Trigger point release	✓ ✓

RECTUS ABDOMINIS

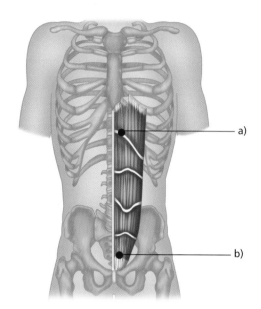

a)

b)

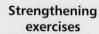

Strengthening exercises

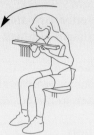

Abdominal machine crunch
(for upper fibres)

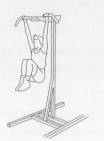

Hanging leg raise

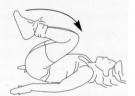

Reverse sit-ups
(for lower fibres)

Self stretches

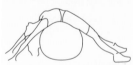

Avoid or take care if you have back problems; check with your health professional first.

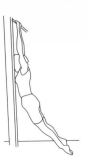

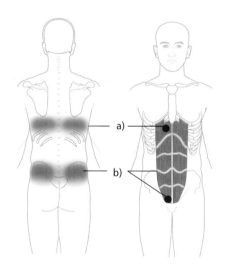

a)

b)

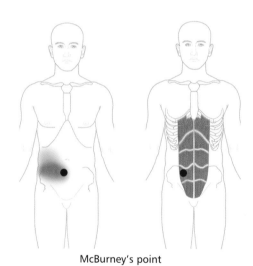

McBurney's point

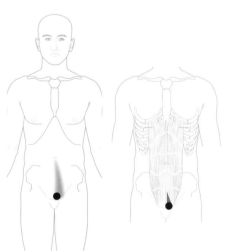

Pyramidalis

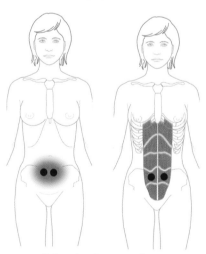

Points for dysmenorrhoea

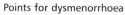

Latin, *rectum*, straight; *abdominis*, belly / stomach.

The rectus abdominis is divided by tendinous bands into three or four bellies, each sheathed in aponeurotic fibres from the lateral abdominal muscles. These fibres converge centrally to form the linea alba. Situated anterior to the lower part of rectus abdominis is a frequently absent muscle called *pyramidalis*, which arises from the pubic crest and inserts into the linea alba. It tenses the linea alba, for reasons unknown.

Origin
Pubic crest and symphysis pubis (front of pubic bone).

Insertion
Anterior surface of xiphoid process. Fifth, sixth and seventh costal cartilages.

Action
Flexes lumbar spine. Depresses ribcage. Stabilizes the pelvis during walking.

Nerve
Ventral rami of thoracic nerves, T5–12.

Basic functional movement
Example: Initiating getting out of a low chair.

Indications
Heartburn. Colic. Dysmenorrhoea. Nausea. Vomiting. Sense of being full. Horizontal back pain.

Referred pain patterns
Upper fibres: horizontal mid back pain; heartburn and indigestion.
Lower fibres: pain between pubis and umbilicus causing dysmenorrhoea.
Lateral fibres: pseudoappendicitis; McBurney's point.

Differential diagnosis
Visceral pathology including; renal, hepatic, pancreatic, diverticular disease, colitis, appendicitis, hiatus hernia, peritoneal disease – pelvic inflammatory disease, ovarian, bladder. Appendicitis. Gynaecological disease. Umbilical / incisional – hernia. Latissimus dorsi.

Advice to patient
Weight.

Techniques

Spray and stretch	✓	✓	Dry needling	✓	✓
Injections	✓	✓	Trigger point release	✓	✓

QUADRATUS LUMBORUM

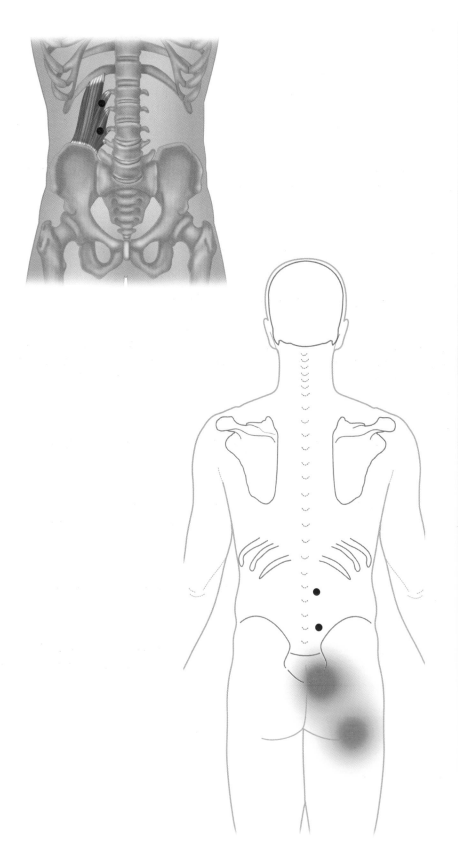

Deep quadratus lumborum

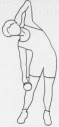

Strengthening exercise

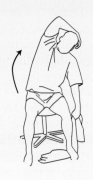

Side bends

Self stretches

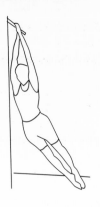

Place towel under left foot. Side bend to left, progressively taking up any slack in towel.

Latin, *quadratus*, squared; *lumbar*, loin.

Origin
Posterior part of iliac crest. Iliolumbar ligament.

Insertion
Medial part of lower border of twelfth rib. Transverse processes of upper four lumbar vertebrae, (L1–L4).

Action
Laterally flexes vertebral column. Fixes the twelfth rib during deep respiration (e.g. helps stabilize the diaphragm for singers exercising voice control). Helps extend lumbar part of vertebral column, and gives it lateral stability.

Nerve
Ventral rami of the subcostal nerve and upper three or four lumbar nerves, T12, L**1**, **2**, **3**.

Basic functional movement
Example: Bending sideways from sitting to pick up an object from the floor.

Indications
Renal tubular acidosis. Discogenic list scoliosis. Mechanical low back pain. Walking stick / cast for fracture. Hip and buttock pain. Greater trochanteric pain (on sleep). Pain turning in bed. Pain standing upright. Persistent deep lower backache at rest. Pain on coughing and sneezing (Valsalva's manoeuvre). Pain on sexual intercourse.

Referred pain patterns
Several 'zones' of pain at; lower abdomen, sacroiliac joint (upper pole), lower buttock, upper hip, and greater trochanter.

Differential diagnosis
Sacroiliitis. Bursitis of hip. Radiculopathy (lumbar). Disc pain (lumbar). Ligamentous pain (iliolumbar and lumbosacral). Spondylosis. Spondyloarthropathy. Stenosis (spinal). Spondylolisthesis. Rib dysfunction (lower).

Also consider
Gluteus medius. Gluteus minimus. Gluteus maximus. Tensor fasciae latae. Pyramidalis. Iliopsoas. Pelvic floor. Sciatica. Hernia. Testicular / scrotal.

Advice to patient
Correct any leg length discrepancy. Change mattress. Occupational advice (mechanical). Hobbies (gardening). Strengthen abdominal (core) stability. Avoid leaning on one leg. Take care when twisting. Emotional component.

Techniques

| Spray and stretch | ✓ | ✓ | Dry needling | | |
| Injections | ✓ | | Trigger point release | ✓ | ✓ |

ILIOPSOAS (PSOAS MAJOR / ILIACUS)

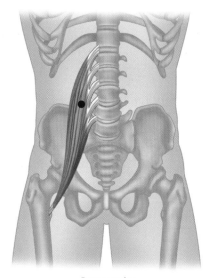

Psoas major

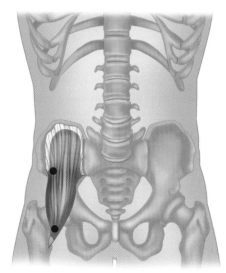

Iliacus

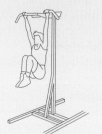

Strengthening exercises

Hanging leg raise

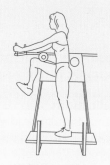

Multi-hip machine
(hip joint flexion)

Self stretches

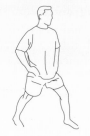

Push right hip forward to
stretch right iliopsoas.
Keep low back flat and
maintain upright posture.

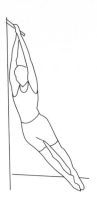

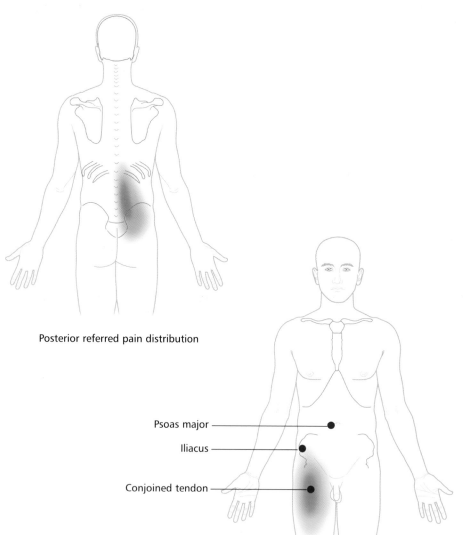

Posterior referred pain distribution

Psoas major —————
Iliacus —————
Conjoined tendon —————

Greek, *psoas*, muscle of loin; *major*, large; *iliacus*, pertaining to the loin.

The psoas major and iliacus are considered part of the posterior abdominal wall due to their position and cushioning role for the abdominal viscera. However, based on their action of flexing the hip joint, it would also be relevant to place them with the hip muscles. Note that some upper fibres of psoas major may insert by a long tendon into the iliopubic eminence to form the psoas minor, which has little function and is absent in about 40% of people. Bilateral contracture of this muscle will increase lumbar lordosis.

Origin
Psoas major: bases of transverse processes of all lumbar vertebrae, (L1–L5). Bodies of twelfth thoracic and all lumbar vertebrae, (T12–L5). Intervertebral discs above each lumbar vertebra.
Iliacus: superior two-thirds of iliac fossa. Internal lip of iliac crest. Ala of sacrum and anterior ligaments of the lumbosacral and sacroiliac joints.

Insertion
Psoas major: lesser trochanter of femur.
Iliacus: lateral side of tendon of psoas major, continuing into lesser trochanter of femur.

Action
Main flexor of hip joint (flexes and laterally rotates thigh, as in kicking a football). Acting from its insertion, flexes the trunk, as in sitting up from the supine position.

Nerve
Psoas major: ventral rami of lumbar nerves, L1, **2**, **3**, 4. (psoas minor innervated from L**1**, **2**).
Iliacus: femoral nerve, L1, **2**, **3**, 4.

Basic functional movement
Example: Going up a step or walking up an incline.

Indications
Low back pain. Groin pain. Increased (hyper) lordosis of lumbar spine. Anterior thigh pain. Pain prominent in lying to sitting up. Scoliosis. Asymmetry (pelvic).

Referred pain patterns
a) Strong vertical ipsilateral paraspinal pain along lumbar spine, diffusely radiating laterally 3–7cm; b) strong zone of pain 5–8cm top of anterior thigh, within diffuse zone from ASIS to upper half of thigh.

Differential diagnosis
Osteoarthritis of hip. Appendicitis. Femoral neuropathy. Meralgia paresthetica. L4–5 disc. Bursitis. Quadriceps muscle injury. Mechanical back dysfunction. Hernia (inguinal / femoral). Gastrointestinal. Rheumatoid arthritis. Space occupying lesions.

Also consider
Quadratus lumborum. Multifidis. Erector spinae. Quadriceps. Hip rotators. Pectineus. Tensor fasciae latae. Adductors (longus and brevis). Femoropatellar joint. Diaphragm.

Advice to patient
Avoid prolonged sitting. Avoid sleeping in foetal position. Treat low back. Avoid overuse in sit ups. Strengthen transversus abdominis. Stretching exercises.

Techniques

| Spray and stretch | ✓ | ✓ | Dry needling | | |
| Injections | ✓ | | Trigger point release | ✓ | ✓ |

7

Muscles of the Shoulder and Upper Arm

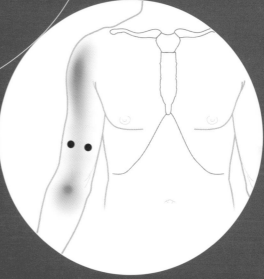

TRAPEZIUS

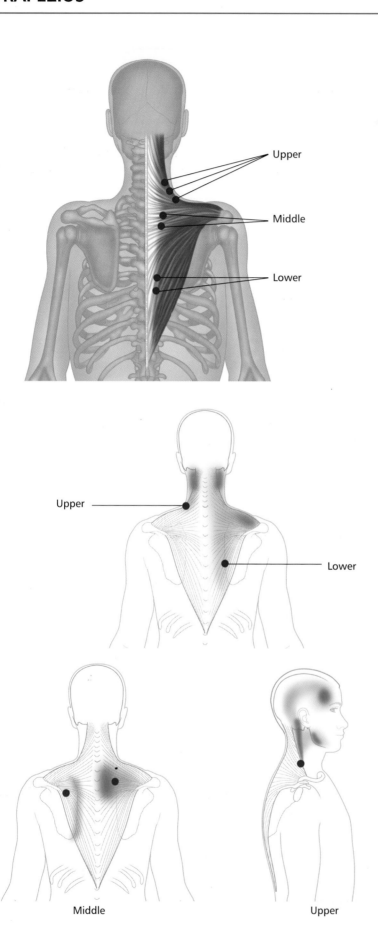

Upper

Middle

Lower

Upper

Lower

Middle

Upper

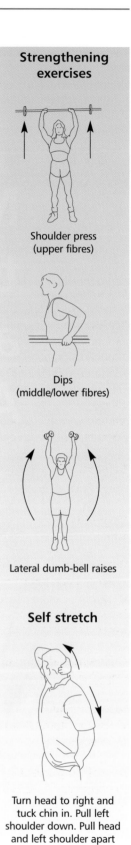

Strengthening exercises

Shoulder press
(upper fibres)

Dips
(middle/lower fibres)

Lateral dumb-bell raises

Self stretch

Turn head to right and
tuck chin in. Pull left
shoulder down. Pull head
and left shoulder apart
from each other.

Latin, *trapezoides*, table shaped.

The left and right trapezius viewed as a whole create a trapezium in shape, thus giving this muscle its name.

Origin
Medial third of superior nuchal line of occipital bone. External occipital protuberance. Ligamentum nuchae. Spinous processes and supraspinous ligaments of seventh cervical vertebra, (C7) and all thoracic vertebrae, (T1–T12).

Insertion
Posterior border of lateral third of clavicle. Medial border of acromion. Upper border of the crest of the spine of scapula, and the tubercle on this crest.

Action
Upper fibres: pull the shoulder girdle up (elevation). Helps prevent depression of the shoulder girdle when a weight is carried on the shoulder or in the hand.
Middle fibres: retract (adduct) scapula.
Lower fibres: depress scapula, particularly against resistance, as when using the hands to get up from a chair.
Upper and lower fibres together: rotate scapula, as in elevating the arm above the head.

Nerve
Motor supply: accessory **X1** nerve.
Sensory supply (proprioception): ventral ramus of cervical nerves, C2, **3**, **4**.

Basic functional movement
Example (upper and lower fibres working together): Painting a ceiling.

Indications
Chronic tension and neck ache. Stress headache. Cervical spine pain. Whiplash.

Referred pain patterns
Upper fibres: pain and tenderness, posterior and lateral aspect of upper neck. Temporal region and angle of jaw.
Middle fibres: local pain radiating medially to spine.
Lower fibres: posterior cervical spine, mastoid area, area above spine of scapula.

Differential diagnosis
Capsular-ligamentous apparatus. Articular dysfunction (facet).

Also consider
Overlap: sternocleidomastoideus. Masseter. Temporalis. Occipitalis. Levator scapulae. Semispinalis. Iliocostalis.

Advice to patient
Posture standing and at work. Stress management. Bra straps. Pectoralis minor tension (round shoulders).

Techniques

| Spray and stretch | ✓ | ✓ | Dry needling | ✓ | ✓ |
| Injections | ✓ | ✓ | Trigger point release | ✓ | ✓ |

LEVATOR SCAPULAE

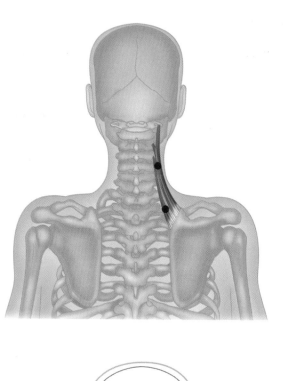

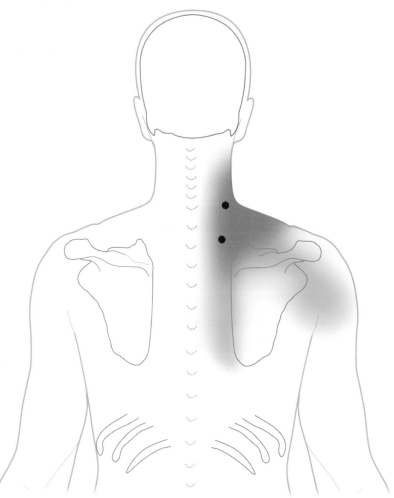

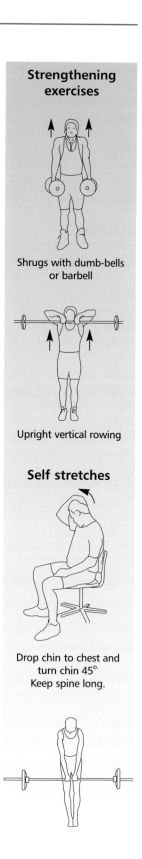

Strengthening exercises

Shrugs with dumb-bells or barbell

Upright vertical rowing

Self stretches

Drop chin to chest and turn chin 45°. Keep spine long.

Latin, *levare*, to lift; *scapulae*, shoulder, blade(s).

Levator scapulae is deep to sternocleidomastoideus and trapezius. It is named after its action of elevating the scapula.

Origin
Posterior tubercles of the transverse processes of the first three or four cervical vertebrae, (C1–C4).

Insertion
Medial (vertebral) border of the scapula between the superior angle and the spine of scapula.

Action
Elevates scapula. Helps retract scapula. Helps bend neck laterally.

Nerve
Dorsal scapular nerve, C**4**, **5** and cervical nerves, C**3**, **4**.

Basic functional movement
Example: Carrying a heavy bag.

Indications
Stiff and painful neck with limited rotation of cervical spine. Long-term use of walking stick.

Referred pain patterns
Triangular pattern from top of scapula to nape of neck. Slight overspill to medial border of scapula and posterior glenohumeral joint.

Differential diagnosis
Scapulothoracic joint dysfunction; winging of scapula. Apophysitis and capsular ligamentous apparatus. Shoulder impingement syndromes.

Also consider
Trapezius. Rhomboids. Splenius cervicis. Erector spinae.

Advice to patient
Holding a telephone shoulder to ear. Stress. Occupation. Air conditioning. Passive stretching. Heat and warmth. Scarf. Change walking stick position.

Techniques

Spray and stretch	✓	✓	Dry needling	✓	✓
Injections	✓	✓	Trigger point release	✓	✓

RHOMBOIDEUS (MINOR AND MAJOR)

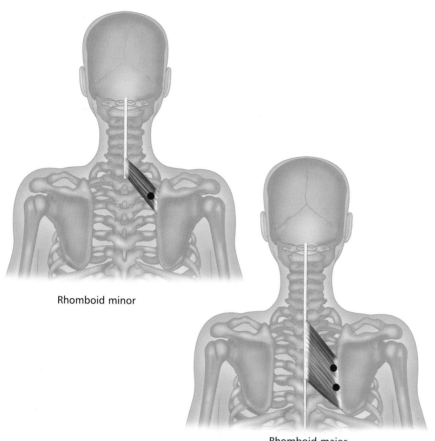

Rhomboid minor

Rhomboid major

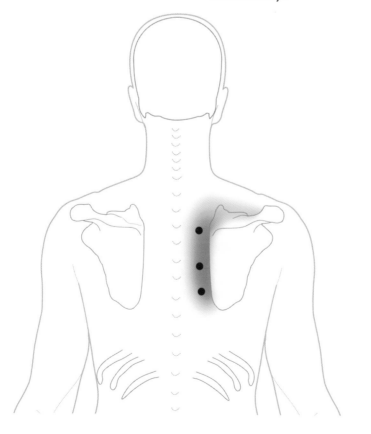

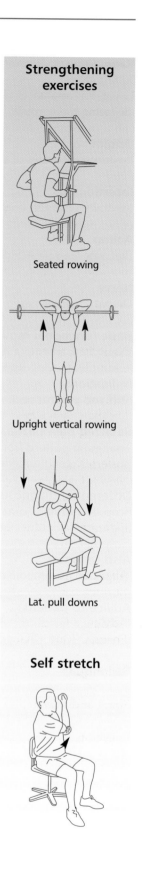

Strengthening exercises

Seated rowing

Upright vertical rowing

Lat. pull downs

Self stretch

Greek, *rhomb*, a parallelogram with oblique angles and only the opposite sides equal; *minor*, small; *major*, large.

So named because of its shape.

Origin
Spinous processes of the seventh cervical vertebra, and upper five thoracic vertebrae, (C7–T1).

Insertion
Medial (vertebral) border of scapula.

Action
Retracts (adducts) scapula. Stabilizes scapula. Slightly assists in outer range of adduction of arm (i.e. from arm overhead to arm at shoulder level).

Nerve
Dorsal scapular nerve, C**4**, **5**.

Basic functional movement
Example: Pulling something towards you, such as opening a drawer.

Indications
Localized pain or chronic aching (C7–T5) region – medial or peri-scapular. Scapulothoracic joint grinding / grating or crunching.

Referred pain patterns
Medial border of scapula, wrapping around superior aspect of spine of scapula towards the acromion process.

Differential diagnosis
Scapulocostal syndrome. Fibromyalgia.

Also consider
Levator scapulae. Middle trapezius. Infraspinatus. Scalenes. Latissimus dorsi.

Advice to patient
Posture. Tight pectoralis muscles. 'Round shoulders'. Occupational posture.

Techniques

Spray and stretch	✓	✓	Dry needling	✓ ✓
Injections	✓		Trigger point release (N.B. pleural cavity)	✓ ✓

SERRATUS ANTERIOR

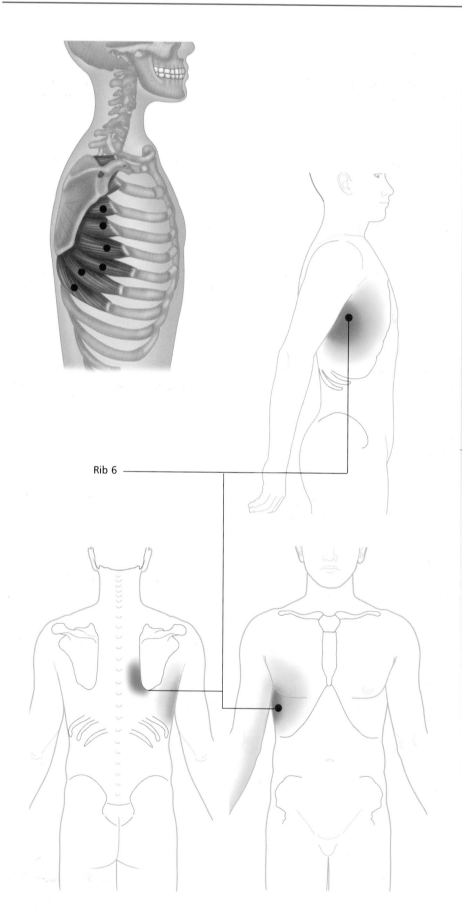

Rib 6

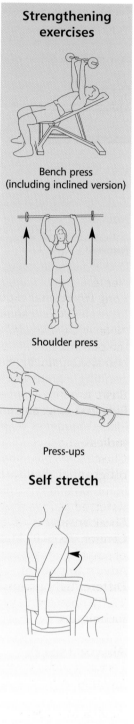

Strengthening exercises

Bench press (including inclined version)

Shoulder press

Press-ups

Self stretch

Latin, *serratus*, serrated; *anterior*, before.

The serratus anterior forms the medial wall of the axilla, along with the upper five ribs. It is a large muscle composed of a series of finger like slips. The lower slips interdigitate with the origin of the external oblique.

Origin
Outer surfaces and superior borders of upper eight or nine ribs, and the fascia covering their intercostal spaces.

Insertion
Anterior (costal) surface of the medial border of scapula and inferior angle of scapula.

Action
Rotates scapula for abduction and flexion of arm. Protracts scapula (pulls it forward on the chest wall and holds it closely in to the chest wall), facilitating pushing movements such as press-ups or punching.

Nerve
Long thoracic nerve, C**5**, **6**, **7**, 8.

Note: A lesion of the long thoracic nerve will result in the medial border of the scapula falling away from the posterior chest wall; resulting in a 'winged scapula' (looking like an angel's wing). A weak muscle will also produce a winged scapula, especially when holding a weight in front of the body.

Basic functional movement
Example: Reaching forwards for something barely within reach.

Indications
Chest pain which does not abate with rest. Breast pain and sensitivity. Panic attacks. Dyspnoea. Chronic cough. Asthma. Renal tubular acidosis. Scapula winging. Chronic 'stitch' on running. Stress.

Referred pain patterns
Local: where each digitation attaches to rib.
Central: rib (6–8), localized pain radiating anterior and posterior in a 5–10cm patch. Pain inferior angle of scapula. Pain in ulnar aspect of the upper extremity.

Differential diagnosis
T7/T8 intercostal nerve entrapment. Herpes zoster. Local vertebral alignment. Rib lesions. Breast pathologies. Reflex-sympathetic dystrophy.

Also consider
Pectoralis major. Sternocleidomastoideus. Scalenus medius. Trapezius. Rhomboideus. Diaphragm. External oblique.

Advice to patient
Avoid cars with heavy steering. Take care with weight-training, especially press ups and bench press. Avoid stress. Try meditation / relaxation.

Techniques

| Spray and stretch | ✓ | ✓ | Dry needling | ✓ | ✓ |
| Injections | ✓ | ✓ | Trigger point release | ✓ | ✓ |

PECTORALIS MAJOR

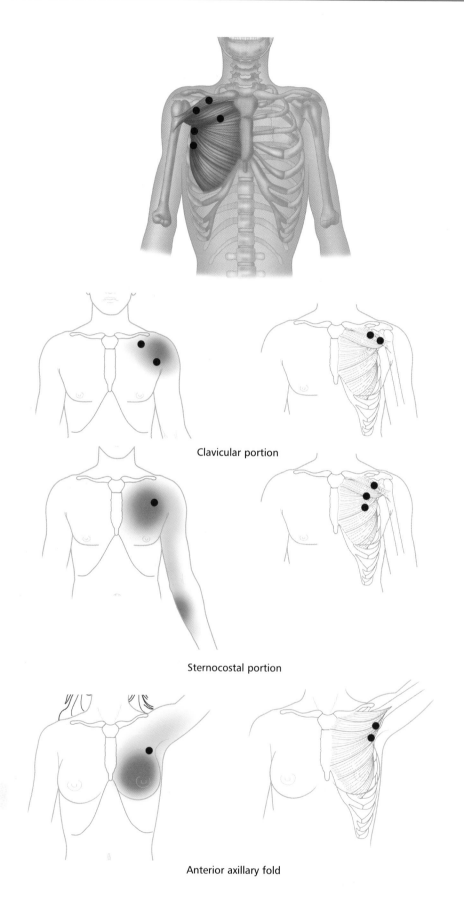

Clavicular portion

Sternocostal portion

Anterior axillary fold

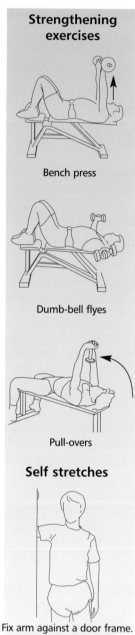

Strengthening exercises

Bench press

Dumb-bell flyes

Pull-overs

Self stretches

Fix arm against a door frame. Step forward keeping your back lengthened, not arched. Raising or lowering arm will stretch different parts of the muscle.

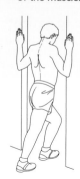

Latin, *pectoralis*, chest; *major*, large.

Along with pectoralis minor, pectoralis major forms the anterior wall of the axilla.

Origin
Clavicular head: medial half or two thirds of front of clavicle.
Sternocostal portion: front of manubrium and body of sternum. Upper six costal cartilages. Rectus sheath.

Insertion
Crest below greater tubercle of humerus. Lateral lip of intertubercular sulcus (bicipital groove) of humerus.

Action
Adducts and medially rotates the humerus.
Clavicular portion: flexes and medially rotates the shoulder joint, and horizontally adducts the humerus towards the opposite shoulder.
Sternocostal portion: obliquely adducts the humerus towards the opposite hip.
The pectoralis major is one of the main climbing muscles, pulling the body up to the fixed arm.

Nerve
Nerve to upper fibres: lateral pectoral nerve, C**5**, **6**, **7**.
Nerve to lower fibres: lateral and medial pectoral nerves, C**6**, **7**, **8**, T**1**.

Basic functional movement
Clavicular portion: brings arm forwards and across the body, e.g. as in applying deodorant to opposite armpit.
Sternocostal portion: pulling something down from above, e.g. such as a rope in bell ringing.

Indications
Post myocardial infarct rehabilitation. Cardiac arrhythmia. Mid-scapular back pain. Breast pain and hypersensitivity. Thoracic outlet syndrome. Anterior shoulder pain. Golfer's and tennis elbow.

Referred pain patterns
Clavicular portion: local pain radiating to the anterior deltoid and long head of biceps brachii area.
Sternal portion: 'acute' back pain into anterior chest wall in a 10–20cm patch of diffuse pain around the medial border of the upper extremity. Stronger pain below medial epicondyle in a 5cm patch, diffuse pain into the 4th and 5th digits.
Costal portion: 5–6th ribs leads to severe cardiac referral (even at night). Intense breast pain (10–15cm patch). Diffuse radiations into axillary tail, and into axilla.

Differential diagnosis
C5–C6 radiculopathy. Biceps tendonitis. Rotator cuff muscle lesions. Intrathoracic pathology. Oesophageal pathology. Tietze's syndrome. Ischaemic heart disease (angina). Thoracic outlet syndrome.

Also consider
Latissimus dorsi. Subscapularis. Teres minor. Infraspinatus. Trapezius (middle fibres). Serratus anterior.

Advice to patient
Round shouldered posture leads to shortening. Work sitting posture is key. Sleeping posture, especially hands folded over chest or hands above head. Bra type and support may be relevant.

Techniques

Spray and stretch	✓	✓	Dry needling	✓	✓
Injections	✓	✓	Trigger point release	✓	✓

LATISSIMUS DORSI

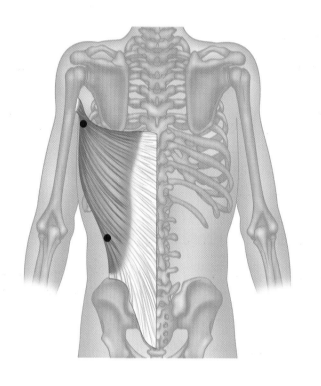

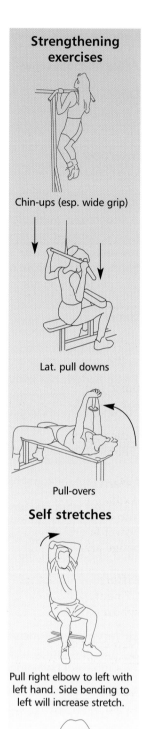

Strengthening exercises

Chin-ups (esp. wide grip)

Lat. pull downs

Pull-overs

Self stretches

Pull right elbow to left with left hand. Side bending to left will increase stretch.

From kneeling on all fours, sit back onto your ankles, keeping your hands fixed. Relax into it and hold for up to two minutes.

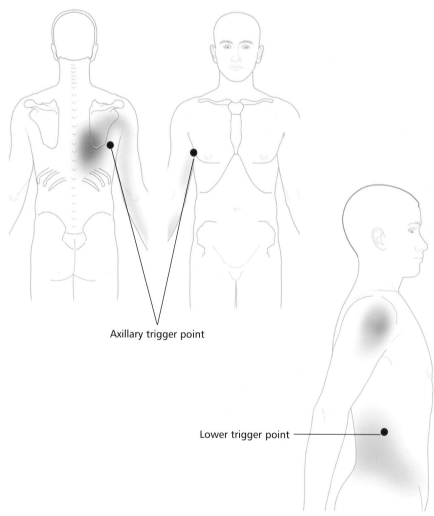

Axillary trigger point

Lower trigger point

Latin, *latissimus*, widest; *dorsi*, of the back.

Along with subscapularis and teres major, the latissimus dorsi forms the posterior wall of the axilla.

Origin
Thoracolumbar fascia, which is attached to the spinous processes of lower six thoracic vertebrae and all the lumbar and sacral vertebrae, (T7–S5) and to the intervening supraspinous ligaments. Posterior part of iliac crest. Lower three or four ribs. Inferior angle of the scapula.

Insertion
Floor of the intertubercular sulcus (bicipital groove) of humerus.

Action
Extends the flexed arm. Adducts and medially rotates the humerus.

It is one of the chief climbing muscles, since it pulls the shoulders downwards and backwards, and pulls the trunk up to the fixed arms (therefore, also active in crawl swimming stroke). Assists in forced inspiration, by raising the lower ribs.

Nerve
Thoracodorsal nerve, C**6**, **7**, **8**, from the posterior cord of the brachial plexus.

Basic functional movement
Example: Pushing on arms of chair to stand up.

Indications
'Thoracic' back pain; constant in nature and unrelated to activity.

Referred pain patterns
Axillary trigger point: a 5–10cm zone of pain at the inferior angle of scapula with diffuse pain radiating into the medial upper extremity into ulnar aspect of hand.
Lower lateral trigger point: triangular pattern from trigger point into the brim of pelvis and regimental badge area.

Differential diagnosis
C7 neuropathy. Ulnar neuropathy. Subscapular nerve entrapment. Axillary neuropathy. Thoracic outlet syndrome. Cardiopulmonary diseases.

Also consider
Rhomboideus. Trapezius (middle fibres). Teres major. Scalenes. Subscapularis. Iliocostalis. Serratus anterior.

Advice to patient
Avoid overloading, e.g. pulling objects down from above head.

Techniques

Spray and stretch	✓	✓	Dry needling	✓	✓
Injections	✓	✓	Trigger point release	✓	✓

DELTOIDEUS

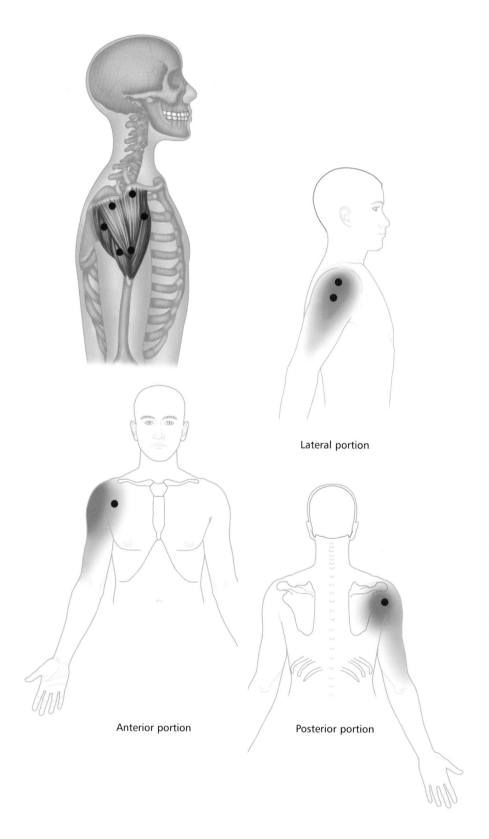

Lateral portion

Anterior portion

Posterior portion

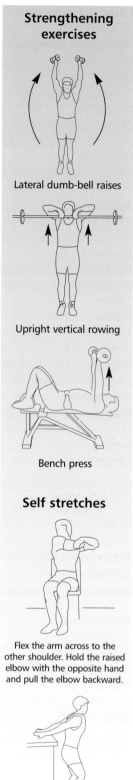

Strengthening exercises

Lateral dumb-bell raises

Upright vertical rowing

Bench press

Self stretches

Flex the arm across to the other shoulder. Hold the raised elbow with the opposite hand and pull the elbow backward.

Keep your arms and torso straight and slowly bend your knees.

Greek, *delta*, fourth letter of Greek alphabet (shaped like a triangle).

The deltoid is composed of three parts; anterior, middle and posterior. Only the middle part is multipennate, probably because its mechanical disadvantage of abduction of the shoulder joint requires extra strength.

Origin
Clavicle, acromion process, and spine of scapula.

Insertion
Deltoid tuberosity situated half way down the lateral surface of the shaft of the humerus.

Action
Anterior fibres: flex and medially rotate the humerus.
Middle fibres: abduct the humerus at the shoulder joint (only after the movement has been initiated by supraspinatus).
Posterior fibres: extend and laterally rotate the humerus.

Nerve
Axillary nerve, C**5**, **6**, from the posterior cord of the brachial plexus.

Basic functional movement
Examples: Reaching for something out to the side. Raising the arm to wave.

Indications
Post trauma rehabilitation. Shoulder pain. Decreased range of motion, esp. in abduction.

Referred pain patterns
Generally localized to the trigger point and within a 5–10cm zone.

Differential diagnosis
Impingement syndromes. Subacromial bursitis. C5 radiculopathy. Rotator cuff tendinopathy. Osteoarthritis of glenohumeral or acromioclavicular joint.

Also consider
Supraspinatus. Infraspinatus. Biceps brachii. Teres minor. Subscapularis. Pectoralis major (clavicular head).

Advice to patient
Stretching (daily). Drive vehicle with two hands. Examine technique with overhead sports such as tennis.

Techniques

Spray and stretch	✓		Dry needling	✓ ✓
Injections	✓		Trigger point release	✓ ✓

SUPRASPINATUS

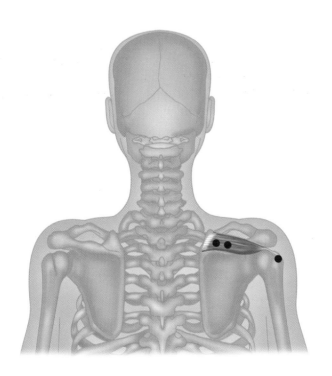

Strengthening exercises

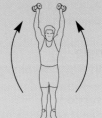

Lateral dumb-bell raises

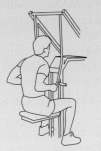

Seated rowing

Self stretch

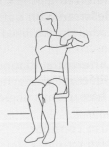

Flex the arm across to the other shoulder. Hold the raised elbow with the opposite hand and pull the elbow backward.

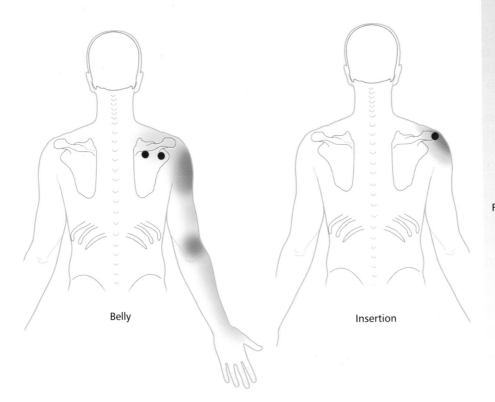

Belly

Insertion

Latin, *supra*, above; *spina*, spine.

A member of the *rotator cuff*, which comprise: *supraspinatus, infraspinatus, teres minor*, and *subscapularis*. The rotator cuff helps hold the head of the humerus in contact with the glenoid cavity (fossa, socket) of the scapula during movements of the shoulder, thus helping to prevent dislocation of the joint.

Origin
Supraspinous fossa of scapula.

Insertion
Upper aspect of the greater tubercle of the humerus. Capsule of shoulder joint.

Action
Initiates the process of abduction at the shoulder joint, so that the deltoid can take over at the later stages of abduction.

Nerve
Suprascapular nerve, C**4**, **5**, **6**, from the upper trunk of the brachial plexus.

Basic functional movement
Example: Holding shopping bag away from side of body.

Indications
Loss of power in abduction. Painful arc syndrome. Night pain / ache. Subacromial bursitis. Rotator cuff tendinopathy.

Referred pain patterns
Belly: deep ache in regimental badge area (4–6cm). Elipse leads to zone of pain in lateral epicondyle / radial head. Diffuse pain into lateral forearm.
Insertion: localized zone of pain 5–8cm over deltoideus.

Differential diagnosis
Phase 1 capsulitis. C5–C6 radiculopathy. Subacromial bursitis (adhesive). Calcific tendonitis. Calcium boils. Rotator cuff tendinopathy.

Also consider
Subscapularis. Infraspinatus. Deltoideus. Trapezius. Latissimus dorsi.

Advice to patient
Avoid heavy carrying. Avoid sleeping with arms above head. Use heat / hot showers.

Techniques

Spray and stretch ✓ ✓   Dry needling ✓

Injections ✓ ✓   Trigger point release ✓ ✓

INFRASPINATUS

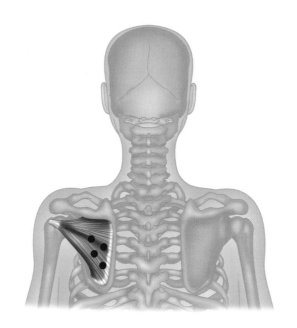

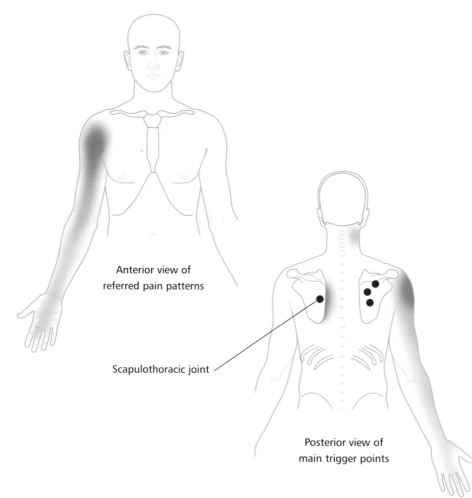

Anterior view of
referred pain patterns

Scapulothoracic joint

Posterior view of
main trigger points

Strengthening exercise

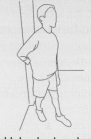

Seated rowing
(limited effect)

Self stretches

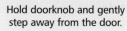

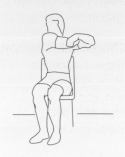

Hold doorknob and gently
step away from the door.

Raise one arm to shoulder
height. Flex the arm across to
the other shoulder. Hold the
raised elbow with the
opposite hand and pull the
elbow backward.

Latin, *infra*, below; *spina*, spine.

A member of the *rotator cuff*, which comprise: *supraspinatus*, *infraspinatus*, *teres minor*, and *subscapularis*. The rotator cuff helps hold the head of the humerus in contact with the glenoid cavity (fossa, socket) of the scapula during movements of the shoulder, thus helping to prevent dislocation of the joint.

Origin
Infraspinous fossa of the scapula.

Insertion
Middle facet on the greater tubercle of humerus. Capsule of shoulder joint.

Action
As a rotator cuff, helps prevent posterior dislocation of the shoulder joint. Laterally rotates humerus.

Nerve
Suprascapular nerve, C(4), **5**, **6**, from the upper trunk of the brachial plexus.

Basic functional movement
Example: Brushing back of hair.

Indications
Decreased range of motion in the Apley's scratch test (behind back). Hemiplegia. Rotator cuff tendinopathy. Frozen shoulder syndrome.

Referred pain patterns
Middle / upper cervical spine: deep anterior shoulder joint zone of 3–4cm in region of long head of biceps brachii radiating into biceps belly, then into forearm – diffuse symptoms in median nerve distribution.
Medial / scapula: to medial border of scapula.

Differential diagnosis
Biceps tendonitis. C5–C6 neuropathy. Suprascapular nerve dysfunction.

Also consider
Infraspinatus. Subscapularis. Levator scapulae. Pectoralis minor / major. Long head of biceps brachii. Biceps brachii. Anterior deltoideus. Teres major. Latissimus dorsi.

Advice to patient
Avoid reaching into back seat of car. Heat can be beneficial. Support arm on pillow for relief.

Techniques

| Spray and stretch | ✓ | ✓ | Dry needling | ✓ | ✓ |
| Injections | ✓ | ✓ | Trigger point release | ✓ | ✓ |

TERES MINOR

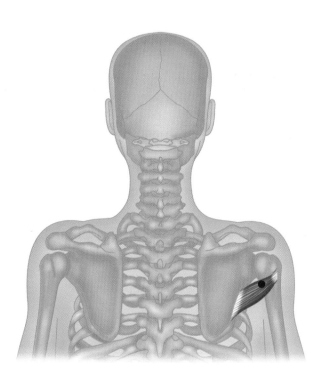

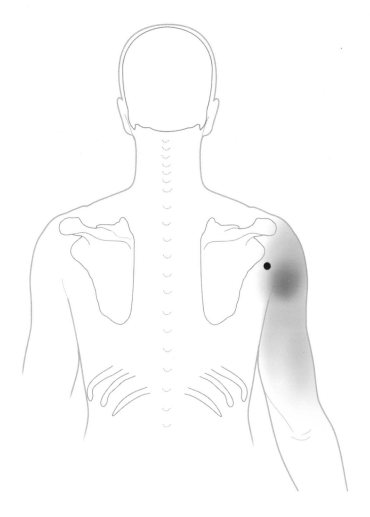

Strengthening exercise

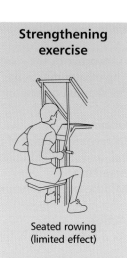

Seated rowing
(limited effect)

Self stretches

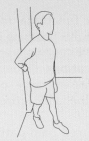

Hold doorknob and gently
step away from the door.

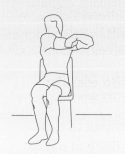

Flex the arm across to
the other shoulder. Hold
the raised elbow with the
opposite hand and pull
the elbow backward.

Latin, *teres*, rounded; finely shaped; *minor*, small.

A member of the *rotator cuff*, which comprise: *supraspinatus*, *infraspinatus*, *teres minor*, and *subscapularis*. The rotator cuff helps hold the head of the humerus in contact with the glenoid cavity (fossa, socket) of the scapula during movements of the shoulder, thus helping to prevent dislocation of the joint.

Origin
Upper two-thirds of the lateral border of the dorsal surface of scapula.

Insertion
Lower facet on the greater tubercle of humerus. Capsule of shoulder joint.

Action
As a rotator cuff, helps prevent upward dislocation of the shoulder joint. Laterally rotates humerus. Weakly adducts humerus.

Nerve
Axillary nerve, C**5**, **6**, from the posterior cord of the brachial plexus.

Basic functional movement
Example: Brushing back of hair.

Indications
Shoulder pain; especially posterior. Frozen shoulder syndrome. Rotator cuff rehabilitation. Subacromial bursitis. Biceps tendonitis.

Referred pain patterns
Localized zone (2–5cm) of intense pain in regimental badge area, with a more diffuse elliptical zone of pain spreading in the postero-lateral upper extremity (above the elbow).

Differential diagnosis
C8–T1 radiculopathy. Rotator cuff tendinopathy. Shoulder-wrist-hand syndrome. Subacromial / deltoid bursitis. Shoulder impingement syndromes (painful arc). Acromioclavicular joint dysfunction.

Also consider
Infraspinatus.

Advice to patient
Posture (round shouldered). Arm position during sleep. Avoid overload. Self stretch.

Techniques

Spray and stretch	✓	✓	Dry needling	✓	✓
Injections	✓	✓	Trigger point release	✓	✓

SUBSCAPULARIS

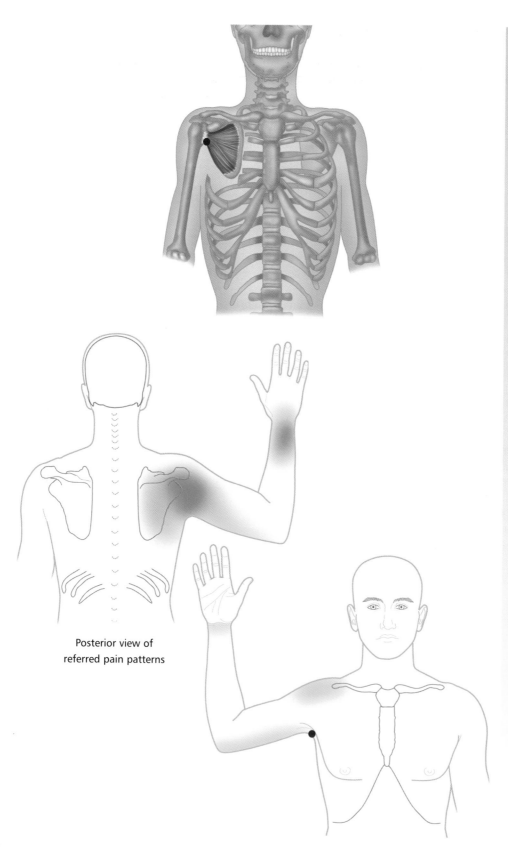

Posterior view of
referred pain patterns

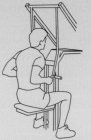

Strengthening exercise

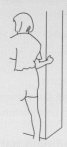

Seated rowing
(limited effect)

Self stretch

Laterally rotate humerus
with elbow bent 90°,
and anchor hand against
door frame.

Latin, *sub*, under; *scapular*, pertaining to the scapula.

A member of the *rotator cuff*, which comprise: *supraspinatus, infraspinatus, teres minor*, and *subscapularis*. The rotator cuff helps hold the head of the humerus in contact with the glenoid cavity (fossa, socket) of the scapula during movements of the shoulder, thus helping to prevent dislocation of the joint. The subscapularis constitutes the greater part of the posterior wall of the axilla.

Origin
Subscapular fossa and the groove along the lateral border of the anterior surface of scapula.

Insertion
Lesser tubercle of humerus. Capsule of shoulder joint.

Action
As a rotator cuff, stabilizes glenohumeral joint; mainly preventing the head of the humerus being pulled upwards by the deltoideus, biceps and long head of triceps. Medially rotates humerus.

Nerve
Upper and lower subscapular nerves, C**5**, **6**, 7, from the posterior cord of the brachial plexus.

Basic functional movement
Example: Reaching into your back pocket.

Indications
Rotator cuff tendinopathy, adhesive capsulitis (frozen shoulder) decreased. Abduction, decreased external rotation.

Referred pain patterns
Axillary trigger point: strong zone (5–8cm) of pain in posterior glenohumeral joint, with a peripheral diffuse zone. Also radiating down posterior aspect of arm and antero-posterior carpals of wrist.

Differential diagnosis
Impingement syndromes. Rotator cuff dysfunctions. Thoracic outlet syndromes. Cervical radiculopathy (C7). Cardiopulmonary pathology.

Also consider
Infraspinatus. Pectoralis minor.

Advice to patient
Round shouldered postures. Walking posture.

Techniques

Spray and stretch	✓ ☐	
Injections	✓ ✓	

Dry needling	✓ ☐	
Trigger point release	✓ ✓	

TERES MAJOR

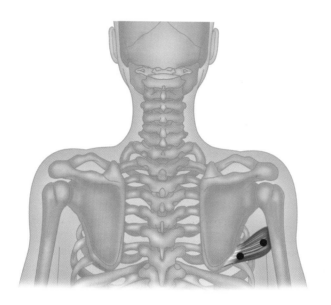

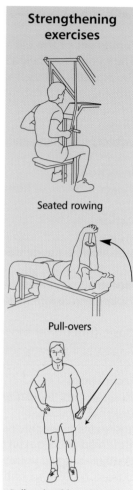

Strengthening exercises

Seated rowing

Pull-overs

Pulley shoulder adduction

Self stretches

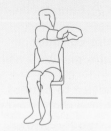

Flex the arm across to the other shoulder. Hold the raised elbow with the opposite hand and pull the elbow backward.

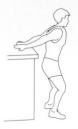

Keep your arms and torso straight and slowly bend your knees.

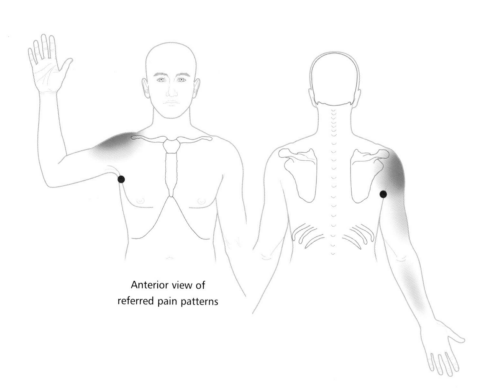

Anterior view of referred pain patterns

Latin, *teres*, rounded, finely shaped; *major*, large.

The teres major, along with the tendon of latissimus dorsi, which passes around it, and the subscapularis, forms the posterior fold of the axilla.

Origin
Oval area on the lower third of the posterior surface of the lateral border of the scapula.

Insertion
Medial lip of the intertubercular sulcus (bicipital groove) of humerus.

Action
Adducts humerus. Medially rotates humerus. Extends humerus from the flexed position.

Nerve
Lower subscapular nerve, C5, **6**, 7, from the posterior cord of the brachial plexus.

Basic functional movement
Example: Reaching into your back pocket.

Indications
Frozen shoulder syndrome. Pain on reaching above the head. Slight pain on rest. Pain when driving. Impingement syndromes.

Referred pain patterns
Deep pain into posterior glenohumeral joint and an oval zone (5–10cm) of pain in posterior deltoid area (can radiate strongly to long head of biceps brachii). Diffuse pain into dorsum of forearm.

Differential diagnosis
Impingement syndromes. Rotator cuff tendinopathy. Cervical neuropatterns (C6–C7). Thoracic outlet syndrome. Supraspinatus calcification.

Also consider
Rhomboideus. Long head of triceps brachii. Latissimus dorsi. Teres minor. Pectoralis minor. Posterior deltoideus.

Advice to patient
Use heat / warmth, especially hot showers. Avoid heavy steering (wheels). Monitor gym activities. Use a pillow at night (to hug). Plenty of self stretching.

Techniques

Spray and stretch	✓ ✓	Dry needling	✓
Injections	✓ ✓	Trigger point release	✓ ✓

BICEPS BRACHII

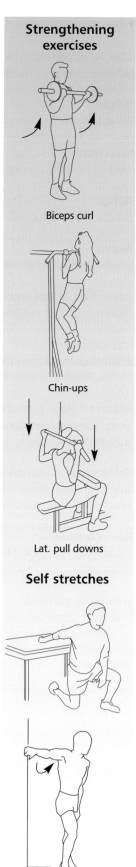

Strengthening exercises

Biceps curl

Chin-ups

Lat. pull downs

Self stretches

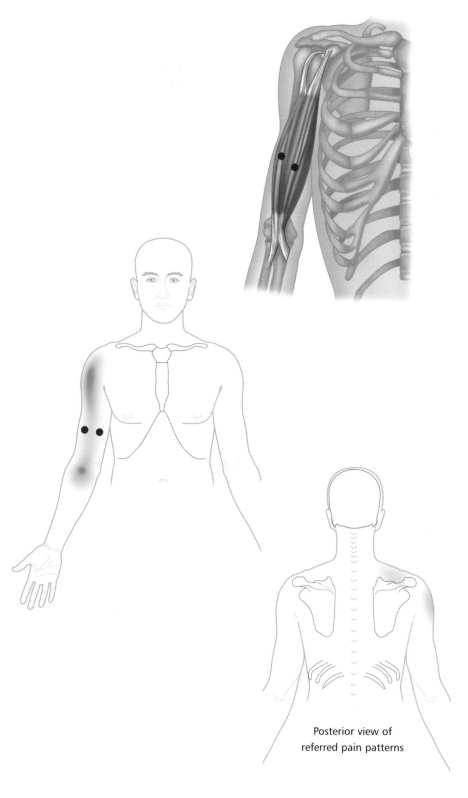

Posterior view of referred pain patterns

Latin, *biceps*, two-headed muscle; *brachii*, of the arm.

Biceps brachii operates over three joints. It has two tendinous heads at its origin and two tendinous insertions. Occasionally it has a third head, originating at the insertion of coracobrachialis. The short head forms part of the lateral wall of the axilla, along with coracobrachialis and the humerus.

Origin
Short head: tip of corocoid process of scapula.
Long head: supraglenoid tubercle of scapula.

Insertion
Posterior part of radial tuberosity.
Bicipital aponeurosis, which leads into the deep fascia on medial aspect of forearm.

Action
Flexes elbow joint. Supinates forearm. (It has been described as the muscle that puts in the corkscrew and pulls out the cork). Weakly flexes arm at the shoulder joint.

Nerve
Musculocutaneous nerve, C**5**, **6**.

Basic functional movement
Examples: Picking up an object. Bringing food to mouth.

Indications
Anterior shoulder pain with decreased arm extension. Biceps tendonitis. Reduced extension of arms. Reduced Apley's scratch test manoeuvre. Frozen shoulder syndrome.

Referred pain patterns
Localized pain with intense ellipse superficially located over the long head tendon. Referred pain into anterior cubital fossa.

Differential diagnosis
Gleno-humeral osteoarthritis. Acromioclavicular osteoarthritis. Supscapularis. Infraspinatus. Subacromial bursitis. Biceps tendonitis. C5 radiculopathy.

Also consider
Subscapularis. Infraspinatus. Brachialis. Supinator. Upper trapezius. Coracobrachialis. Triceps brachii.

Advice to patient
Exercise antagonists (triceps brachii). Reduce load on biceps brachii when carrying with a bent arm. Sleeping position. Work posture.

Techniques

| Spray and stretch | ✓ | ✓ | Dry needling | ✓ | |
| Injections | ✓ | ✓ | Trigger point release | ✓ | ✓ |

TRICEPS BRACHII

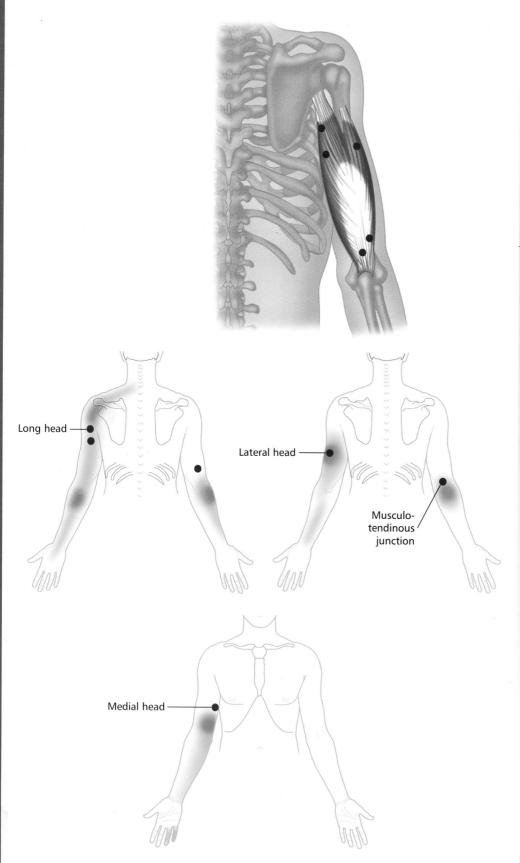

Long head

Lateral head

Musculo-tendinous junction

Medial head

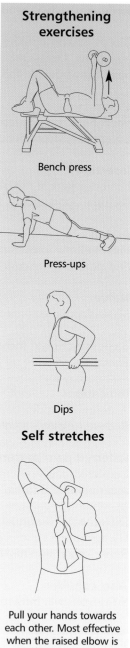

Strengthening exercises

Bench press

Press-ups

Dips

Self stretches

Pull your hands towards each other. Most effective when the raised elbow is against a wall.

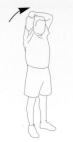

Keep your head up and elbow as far back as is comfortable, without hollowing your lower back.

Latin, *triceps*, three-headed muscle; *brachii*, of the arm.

The triceps originates from three heads and is the only muscle on the back of the arm.

Origin
Long head: infraglenoid tubercle of the scapula.
Lateral head: upper half of posterior surface of shaft of humerus (above and lateral to the radial groove).
Medial head: lower half of posterior surface of shaft of humerus (below and medial to the radial groove).

Insertion
Posterior part of the olecranon process of the ulna.

Action
Extends (straightens) elbow joint. Long head can adduct the humerus and extend it from the flexed position. Stabilizes shoulder joint.

Nerve
Radial nerve, C6, **7**, **8**, T1.

Basic functional movement
Examples: Throwing objects. Pushing a door shut.

Indications
Golfer's elbow. Tennis elbow. Arthritis of elbow and / or shoulder. Chronic use of crutches / walking stick. Repetitive mechanical activities of arms. Raquet sports.

Referred pain patterns
a) Long head: pain at supero-lateral border of shoulder radiating diffusely down posterior upper extremity with a strong zone of pain around olecranon process, and then vaguely into the posterior forearm; b) medial head: 5cm patch of pain in medial epicondyle radiating along medial border of forearm to digits 4 and 5; c) lateral head: strong midline pain into upper extremity radiating vaguely into posterior forearm.

Differential diagnosis
Radial nerve injury. Ulnar neuropathy. C7 neuropathy (cervical disc).

Also consider
Teres minor. Teres major. Latissimus dorsi. Anconeus. Supinator. Brachioradialis. Extensor carpi radialis longus.

Advice to patient
Review arm positions on repetitive manual work. Take regular breaks. New tennis raquet or widen grip. Avoid overhead activities.

Techniques

Spray and stretch	✓	✓	Dry needling	✓	
Injections	✓	✓	Trigger point release	✓	✓

8

Muscles of the Forearm and Hand

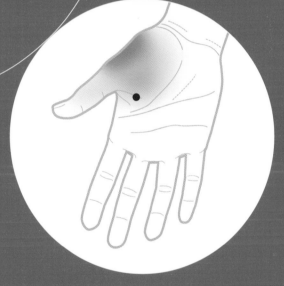

PRONATOR TERES

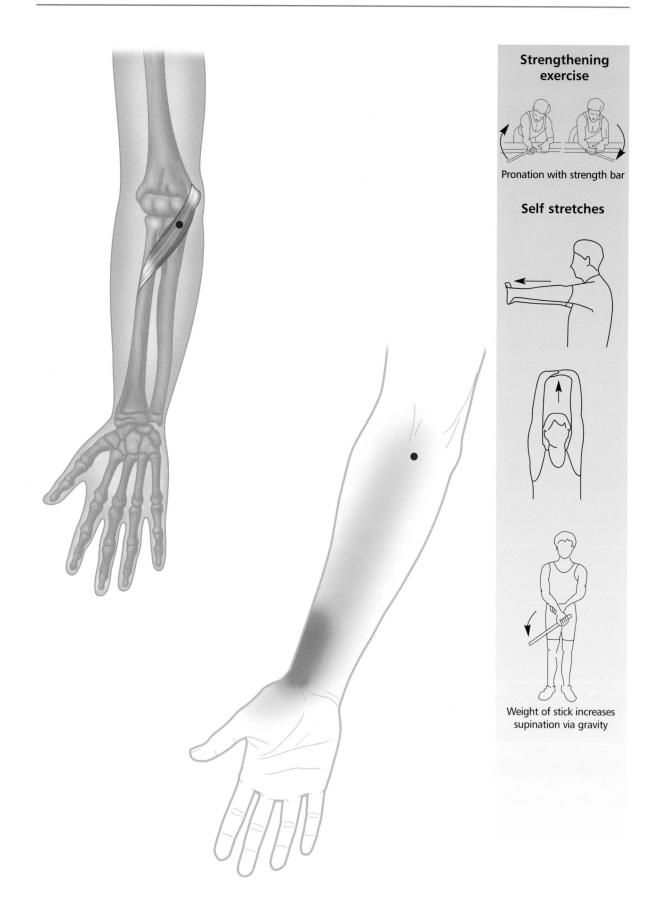

Strengthening exercise

Pronation with strength bar

Self stretches

Weight of stick increases supination via gravity

Latin, *pronate*, bent forward; *teres*, rounded, finely shaped.

Origin
Humeral head: lower third of medial supracondylar ridge and the common flexor origin on the anterior aspect of the medial epicondyle of humerus.
Ulnar head: medial border of the coronoid process of the ulna.

Insertion
Mid-lateral surface of radius (pronator tuberosity).

Action
Pronates forearm. Assists flexion of elbow joint.

Nerve
Median nerve, C**6**, 7.

Basic functional movement
Examples: Pouring liquid from a container. Turning a doorknob.

Indications
Pain in wrist (lateral). Pain on supination. Hairdressers (over use of scissors). Inability to 'cup' hands together, esp. 'cupping' and extension of the wrist. Shoulder pain (compensatory). Wrist pain on driving.

Referred pain patterns
Strong pain 'deep' into palmar region of the wrist (lateral) radiating up the antero-lateral forearm.

Differential diagnosis
De Quervain's tenosynovitis. Carpal tunnel swelling. Osteoarthritis of proximal thumb joint. Distal radio-ulnar discopathy. Epicondylitis.

Also consider
Finger flexors. Scalenes. Pectoralis major.

Advice to patient
Stretching techniques. Self massage. Change grip and techniques in tennis / golf. Review driving posture, and grip on steering wheel.

Techniques

Spray and stretch	✓	✓	Dry needling	✓	✓
Injections	✓	✓	Trigger point release	✓	✓

PALMARIS LONGUS

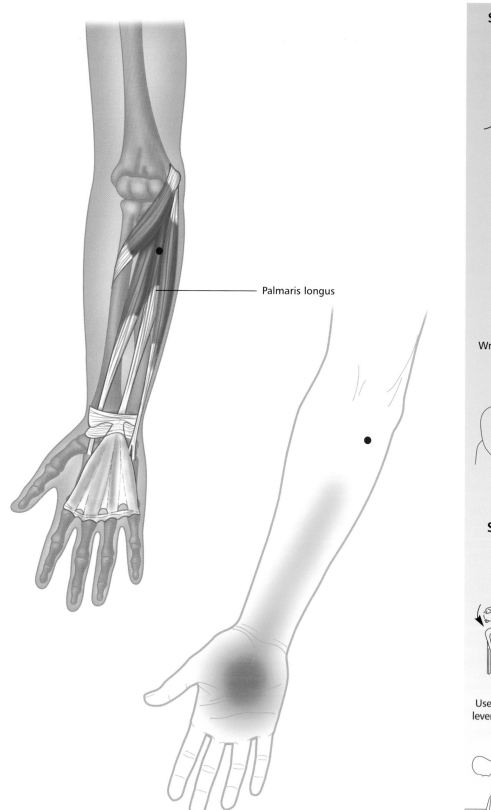

Palmaris longus

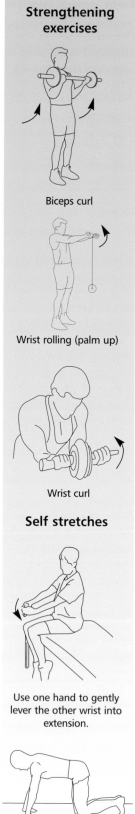

Strengthening exercises

Biceps curl

Wrist rolling (palm up)

Wrist curl

Self stretches

Use one hand to gently lever the other wrist into extension.

Latin, *palmaris*, palma, palm; *longus*, long.

Part of the superficial layer, which also includes: pronator teres, flexor carpi radialis, and flexor carpi ulnaris. The palmaris longus muscle is absent in 13% of the population.

Origin
Common flexor origin on the anterior aspect of the medial epicondyle of humerus.

Insertion
Superficial (front) surface of flexor retinaculum and apex of the palmar aponeurosis.

Action
Flexes the wrist. Tenses the palmar fascia.

Nerve
Median nerve, C(6), **7**, **8**, T1.

Basic functional movement
Examples: Grasping a small ball. Cupping the palm to drink from the hand.

Indications
Pain and 'soreness' in palm of hand. Tenderness in hand / palm. Functional loss of power in grip. Tennis elbow.

Referred pain patterns
Diffuse pain in anterior forearm; intense pain zone 2–3cm in palm of hand surrounded by a superficial zone of prickling and needle-like sensations.

Differential diagnosis
Neurogenic pain. Dupuytren's contracture. Carpal tunnel syndrome. Complex regional pain syndrome (reflex sympathetic dystrophy). Scleroderma. Dermatomyositis.

Also consider
Flexor carpi radialis. Brachialis. Pronator teres. Wrist joints (carpals). Triceps brachii.

Advice to patient
Avoid prolonged 'gripping' especially power tools, often seen in massage therapists. Stretching and heat. Regular breaks.

Techniques

Spray and stretch	✓ ✓	Dry needling	✓ ☐
Injections	✓ ✓	Trigger point release	✓ ✓

WRIST FLEXORS

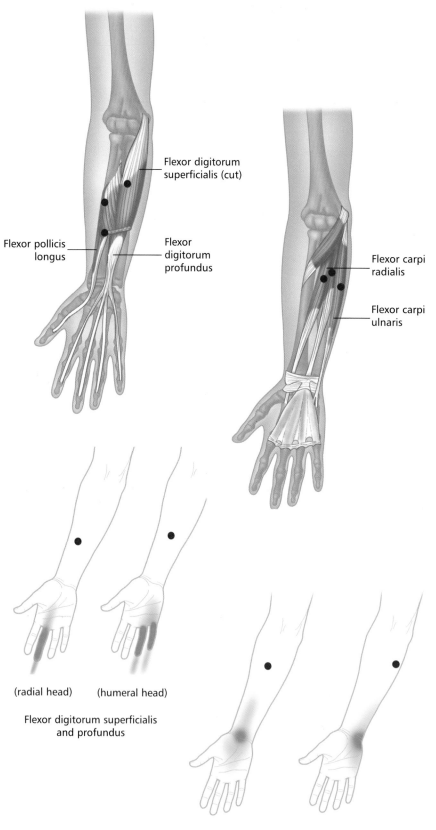

Flexor digitorum superficialis (cut)

Flexor pollicis longus

Flexor digitorum profundus

Flexor carpi radialis

Flexor carpi ulnaris

(radial head)   (humeral head)

Flexor digitorum superficialis and profundus

Flexor carpi radialis   Flexor carpi ulnaris

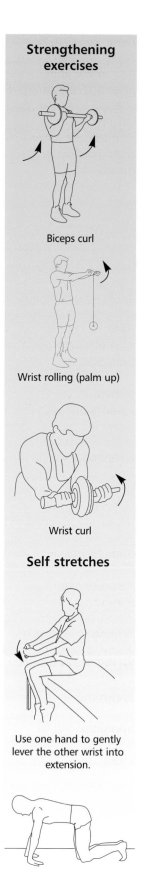

Strengthening exercises

Biceps curl

Wrist rolling (palm up)

Wrist curl

Self stretches

Use one hand to gently lever the other wrist into extension.

Latin, *flex*, to bend; *carpi*, of the wrist; *radius*, staff, spoke of wheel; *ulnaris*, of the elbow / arm; *digit*, finger; *superficialis*, on the surface; *profundus*, deep.

Flexor carpi radialis, flexor carpi ulnaris, flexor digitorum superficialis, and flexor digitorum profundus.

Origin
Common flexor origin on the anterior aspect of the medial epicondyle of humerus (i.e. lower medial end of humerus).

Insertion
Carpals, metacarpals, and phalanges.

Action
Flex the wrist joint. (Flexor carpi radialis also abducts the wrist; flexor carpi ulnaris also adducts the wrist).

Nerve
Median nerve, C6, **7**, **8**, T1.

Basic functional movement
Examples: Pulling rope in towards you. Wielding an axe or hammer. Pouring liquid from bottle. Turning door handle.

Indications
Hand, wrist, and finger pain. Trigger finger. Cutting with scissors. Gripping. Golfer's elbow. Repetitive strain injury. Hairdressers. Turning hand to cupping action. Tense finger flexors.

Referred pain patterns
Individual muscles refer to the lower arm, wrist, hand, and fingers (*see* diagrams).

Differential diagnosis
Ulnar neuritis. Cervical neuropathies. Carpal bone dysfunctions. De Quervain's tenosynovitis. Repetitive strain injury. Osteo- and rheumatoid arthritis. Radio-ulnar disc (distal) problems. Carpal tunnel syndrome. Medial epicondylitis.

Also consider
Shoulder muscles. Upper arm muscles. Scalenes. Flexor pollicis longus.

Advice to patient
Avoid prolonged gripping. Avoid repeated twisting (screwdriver). Change golf grip. Take regular breaks. Regular finger stretching.

Techniques

Spray and stretch	✓	✓	Dry needling	✓	
Injections	✓		Trigger point release	✓	✓

BRACHIORADIALIS

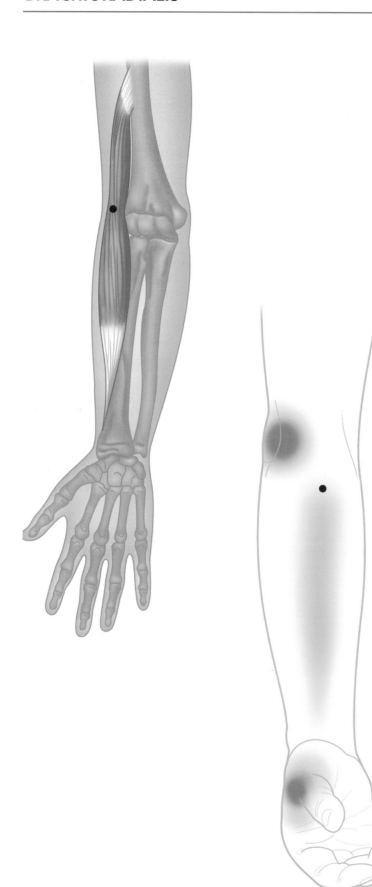

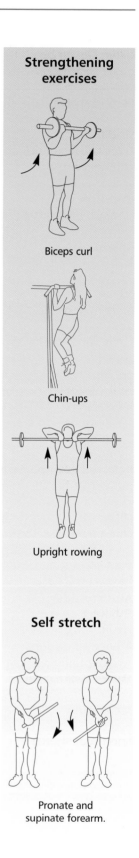

Strengthening exercises

Biceps curl

Chin-ups

Upright rowing

Self stretch

Pronate and supinate forearm.

Latin, *brachial*, relating to the arm; *radius*, staff, spoke of wheel.

Part of the superficial group. The brachioradialis forms the lateral border of the cubital fossa. The muscle belly is prominent when working against resistance.

Origin
Upper two-thirds of the anterior aspect of lateral supracondylar ridge of humerus (i.e. lateral part of shaft of humerus, 5–7.5cm (2–3″) above elbow joint).

Insertion
Lower lateral end of radius, just above the styloid process.

Action
Flexes elbow joint. Assists in pronating and supinating forearm when these movements are resisted.

Nerve
Radial nerve, C**5, 6**.

Basic functional movement
Example: Turning a corkscrew.

Indications
Elbow pain. Pain in thumb (dorsum). Tennis elbow (lateral epicondylitis). Weakness in grip. Repetitive strain injury.

Referred pain patterns
Lateral epicondyle area 3–4cm patch with vague arm pain (radius border), localizing into strong pain dorsum of thumb.

Differential diagnosis
De Quervain's tenosynovitis. Osteoarthritis of thumb (trapezium).

Also consider
Biceps brachiii. Brachialis. Extensor carpi radialis longus, and brevis. Supinator. Extensor digitorum.

Advice to patient
Avoid long standing. Carrying (briefcases). Take regular breaks when typing. Use wrist supports. Change grip on tennis raquet.

Techniques

Spray and stretch	✓	✓	Dry needling	✓	✓
Injections	✓	✓	Trigger point release	✓	✓

WRIST EXTENSORS

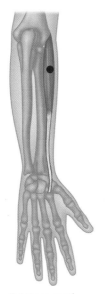

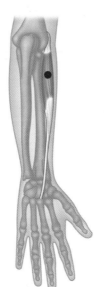

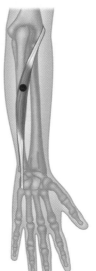

Extensor carpi
radialis longus

Extensor carpi
radialis brevis

Extensor carpi
ulnaris

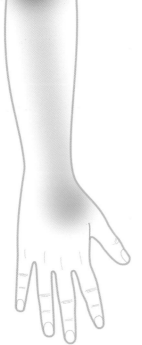

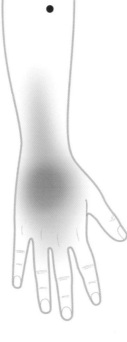

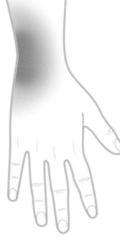

Extensor carpi
radialis longus

Extensor carpi
radialis brevis

Extensor carpi
ulnaris

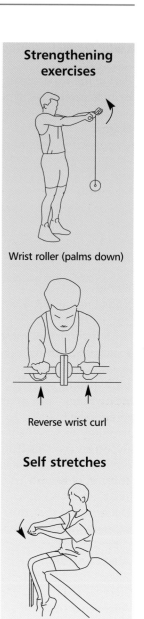

Strengthening exercises

Wrist roller (palms down)

Reverse wrist curl

Self stretches

Use lower hand to gently lever the other wrist into flexion.

Latin, *extensor*, to extend; *carpi*, of the wrist; *radius*, staff, spoke of wheel; *longus*, long; *brevis*, short; *ulnaris*, of the elbow.

Includes extensor carpi radialis longus and brevis, and extensor carpi ulnaris.

Origin
Common extensor tendon from lateral epicondyle of humerus (i.e. lower lateral end of humerus).

Insertion
Dorsal surface of metacarpal bones.

Action
Extends the wrist (extensor carpi radialis and brevis also abduct the wrist; extensor carpi ulnaris also adducts the wrist).

Nerve
Radialis longus and brevis: radial nerve, C5, **6**, **7**, 8.
Extensor carpi ulnaris: deep radial (posterior interosseous) nerve, C5, 6, **7**, **8**.

Basic functional movement
Examples: Kneading dough. Typing. Cleaning windows.

Indications
Forearm, elbow, wrist, and hand pain. Finger stiffness. Painful / weak grip. Tennis elbow. Pain on gripping and twisting, seen in musicians / athletes / long distance drivers. Loss of control (fine) on gripping activities.

Referred pain patterns
Extensor carpi radialis longus: strong 2–3cm zone over lateral epicondyle, diffusely radiating to dorsum of hand above thumb.
Extensor carpi radialis brevis: strong zone of pain 3–5cm over dorsum of hand.
Extensor carpi ulnaris: strong localized specific referral to dorsal ulnar surface of hand, and bulk of wrist.

Differential diagnosis
Epicondylitis. C5–C6 radiculopathy. De Quervain's tenosynovitis. Articular dysfunction of wrist. Osteoarthritis. Carpal tunnel syndrome.

Also consider
Supinator. Brachioradialis. Extensor digitorum. Triceps brachii. Biceps brachii. Anconeus.

Advice to patient
Avoid 'over' gripping in sports. Take regular breaks / rests when gardening / driving. Explore occupational factors / ergonomics. Home stretch and exercises. Change grip width in golf / tennis. Use of wrist splints.

Techniques

Spray and stretch	✓	✓	Dry needling	✓	✓
Injections	✓	✓	Trigger point release	✓	

EXTENSOR DIGITORUM

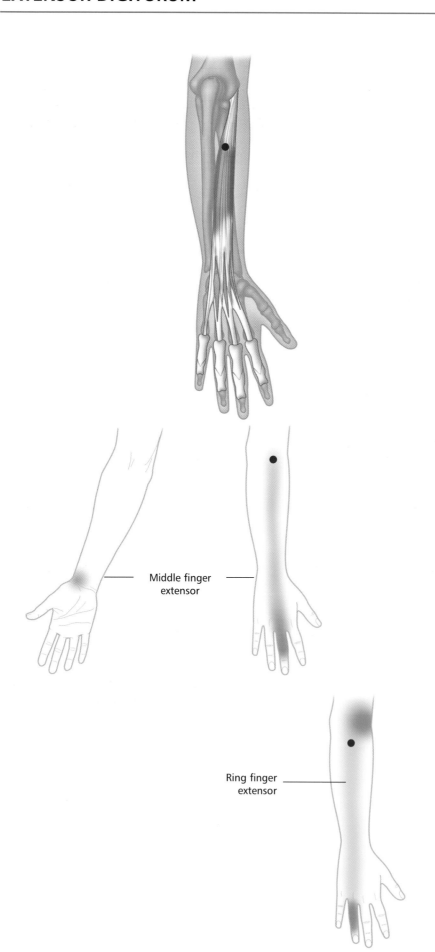

Middle finger extensor

Ring finger extensor

Strengthening exercise

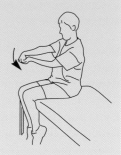

Exer. ring finger extension

Self stretches

Use one hand to gently lever the other wrist and therefore fingers into extension.

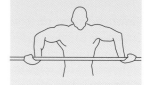

Latin, *extensor*, to extend; *digit*, finger.

Part of the superficial group. Each tendon of extensor digitorum, over each metacarpophalangeal joint, forms a triangular membranous sheet called the *extensor hood* or *extensor expansion*, into which inserts the lumbricales and interossei of the hand. Extensor digiti minimi and extensor indicis also insert into the extensor expansion.

Origin
Common extensor tendon from lateral epicondyle of humerus (i.e. lower lateral end of humerus).

Insertion
Dorsal surfaces of all the phalanges of the four fingers.

Action
Extends the fingers (metacarpophalangeal and interphalangeal joints). Assists abduction (divergence) of fingers away from the middle finger.

Nerve
Deep radial (posterior interosseous) nerve, C**6**, **7**, **8**.

Basic functional movement
Example: Letting go of objects held in the hand.

Indications
Finger, hand, and wrist pain. Elbow pain. Stiffness and pain in fingers. Weakness in fingers (decreased grip). Tennis elbow. Pain on forceful gripping, often seen in professional musicians (esp. guitarists).

Referred pain patterns
Diffuse pain from forearm becoming more intense in the appropriate finger (proximal metacarpal). Pain in lateral epicondyle.

Differential diagnosis
Radiculopathy (cervical). Epicondylitis (tennis elbow). Osteoarthritis of fingers. De Quervain's tenosynovitis. Mechanical wrist pain (carpals).

Also consider
Brachioradialis. Supinator. Extensor carpi radialis longus. Extensor indicis.

Advice to patient
Home exercise programme. Self stretch. Avoid sustained gripping. Explore work posture / arrangement with reference to computer keyboards / mouse. Avoid habitual postures such as sleeping with hands folded under head / pillow.

Techniques

Spray and stretch	✓ ✓	Dry needling ✓ ✓
Injections	✓ ✓	Trigger point release ✓

SUPINATOR

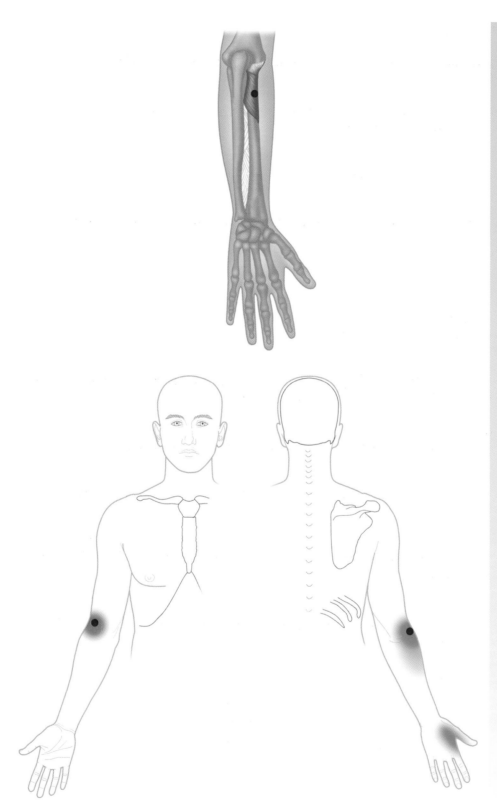

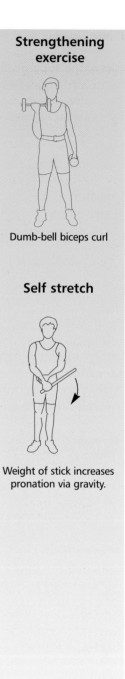

Strengthening exercise

Dumb-bell biceps curl

Self stretch

Weight of stick increases pronation via gravity.

Latin, *supinus*, lying on the back.

Part of the deep group. Supinator is almost entirely concealed by the superficial muscles.

Origin
Lateral epicondyle of humerus. Radial collateral (lateral) ligament of elbow joint. Annular ligament of superior radio-ulnar joint. Supinator crest of ulna.

Insertion
Dorsal and lateral surfaces of upper third of radius.

Action
Supinates forearm (for which it is probably the main prime mover; with biceps brachii being an auxiliary).

Nerve
Deep radial nerve, C5, **6**, (7).

Basic functional movement
Example: Turning a door handle, or screwdriver.

Indications
Tennis elbow. Thumb joint pain. Elbow pain (when carrying and at rest). Pain turning door knobs. Localized pain on supination. Chronic use of walking stick. Pain on handshake.

Referred pain patterns
Localized 3–5cm strong zone of pain at lateral epicondyle and at web of thumb (dorsum).

Differential diagnosis
De Quervain's tenosynovitis. Lateral epicondylitis (tendino-osseous, musculo-tendinous, intramuscular). Radial head dysfunction.

Also consider
Common extensors. Biceps brachii. Triceps brachii (insertion). Anconeus. Brachialis. Palmaris longus. Brachioradialis. Extensor carpi radialis longus.

Advice to patient
Change tennis style (keep wrists dorsiflexed). Change grip size. Avoid prolonged gripping / carrying. Change walking stick side regularly. Use pressure bandage / strap. Use backpack.

Techniques

| Spray and stretch | ✓ | ✓ | Dry needling | ✓ | |
| Injections | ✓ | ✓ | Trigger point release | ✓ | ✓ |

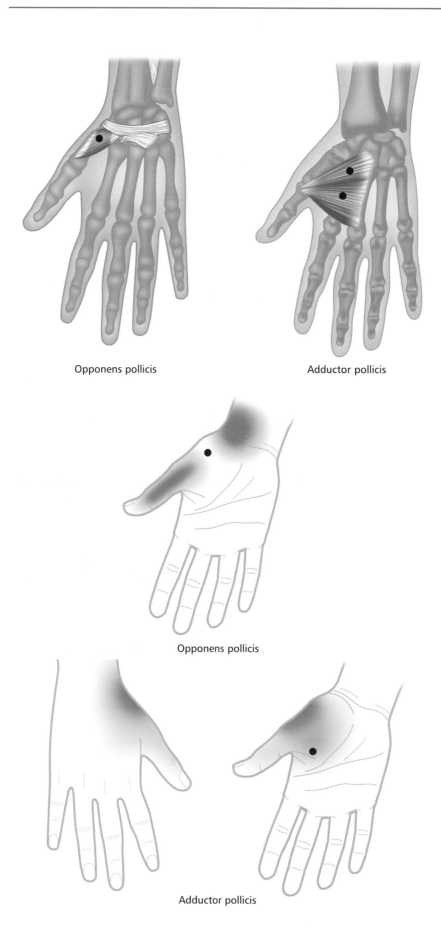

Opponens pollicis

Adductor pollicis

Opponens pollicis

Adductor pollicis

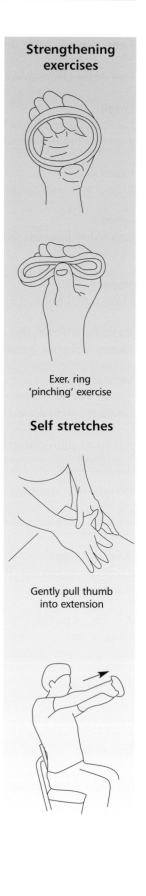

Strengthening exercises

Exer. ring 'pinching' exercise

Self stretches

Gently pull thumb into extension

Latin, *opponens*, opposing; *pollicis*, of the thumb; *adduct*, toward.

Opponens pollicis is part of the thenar eminence, usually partly fused with flexor pollicis brevis and deep to abductor pollicis brevis.

Origin
Opponens pollicis: flexor retinaculum. Tubercle of trapezium.
Adducor pollicis: oblique fibres: anterior surfaces of second and third metacarpals, capitate and trapezoid. Transverse fibres: palmar surface of third metacarpal bone.

Insertion
Opponens pollicis: entire length of radial border of first metacarpal.
Adductor pollicis: ulna (medial) side of base of proximal phalanx of thumb.

Action
Opponens pollicis: opposes (i.e. abducts, then slightly medially rotates, followed by flexion and adduction) the thumb so that the pad of the thumb can be drawn into contact with the pads of the fingers.
Adductor pollicis: adducts the thumb.

Nerve
Opponens pollicis: median nerve, (C6, 7, 8, T1).
Adductor pollicis: deep ulnar nerve, C**8**, T**1**.

Basic functional movement
Example: Picking up small object between thumb and fingers (opponens pollicis). Gripping a jam jar lid to screw it on (adductor pollicis).

Indications
'Weeder's thumb'. Thumb pain on activity. Difficulty on maintaining pincer movement. 'Texter's', and 'video gamer's' thumb. Pain on sewing, writing, and opening jars. Loss of fine motor control in buttoning, sewing, writing, and painting, etc.

Referred pain patterns
Opponens pollicis: palmar wrist pain at distal radial head and into palmar aspect of thumb.
Adductor pollicis: dorsal and palmar surfaces of thumb localized around metacarpophalangeal joint and radiating to web of thumb and thenar eminence.

Differential diagnosis
De Quervain's tenosynovitis. Osteoarthritis of thumb (saddle joint). Rheumatoid arthritis. Carpal tunnel syndrome. 'Trigger thumb'. Discopathy of distal radio-ulnar joint. Carpal bones dysfunction. Mechanical dysfunction. Fracture. Subluxation.

Also consider
Abductor pollicis brevis. Flexor pollicis brevis. Flexor pollicis longus.

Advice to patient
Home stretching exercises. Take regular breaks. Ergonomic pens, etc. Use warmth.

Techniques

Spray and stretch	✓	✓	Dry needling	✓	
Injections	✓	✓	Trigger point release	✓	

SMALL HAND MUSCLES

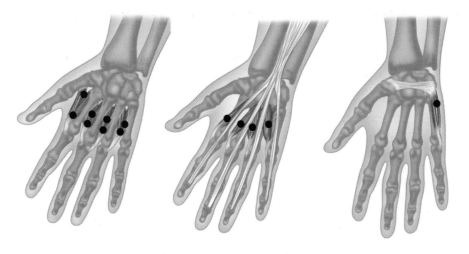

Dorsal interossei   Lumbricales   Abductor digiti minimi

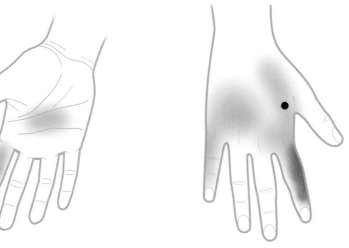

Palmar view   First dorsal interosseous   Dorsal view

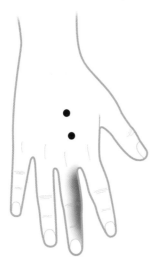

Dorsal view
Second dorsal interosseous

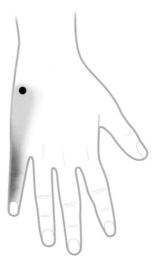

Dorsal view
Abductor digiti minimi

Latin, *dorsal*, back; *interosseus*, between bones; *lumbrical*, earthworm; *abductor*, away from; *digit*, finger; *minimi*, smallest.

Comprising: dorsal interossei, lumbricales, and abductor digiti minimi. The four dorsal interossei are about twice the size of the palmar interossei. The lumbricales compose of small cylindrical muscles, one for each finger. Abductor digiti minimi is the most superficial muscle of the hypothenar eminence.

Origin
Dorsal interossei: by two heads, each from adjacent sides of metacarpals.
Lumbricales: tendons of flexor digitorum profundus in the palm.
Abductor digiti minimi: pisiform bone. Tendon of flexor carpi ulnaris.

Insertion
Dorsal interossei: into the extensor expansion and to base of proximal phalanx.
Lumbricales: lateral (radial) side of corresponding tendon of extensor digitorum, on the dorsum of the respective digits.
Abductor digiti minimi: Ulna (medial) side of base of proximal phalanx of little finger.

Action
Dorsal interossei: abduct fingers away from middle finger. Assist in flexion of fingers at metacarpophalangeal joints.
Lumbricales: extend the interphalangeal joints and simultaneously flex the metacarpophalangeal joints of the fingers.
Abductor digiti minimi: abducts the little finger.

Nerve
Dorsal interossei: ulnar nerve, C**8**, T**1**.
Lumbricales: lateral; median nerve, C(6), 7, **8**, T**1**; medial; ulnar nerve, C(7), **8**, T**1**.
Abductor digiti minimi: ulnar nerve, C(7), **8**, T**1**.

Basic functional movement
Example: Spreading fingers. Cupping your hand. Holding a large ball.

Indications
Finger pain and stiffness. Pain when pinching / gripping, associated with Heberdan's node(s), e.g. in professional musicians (esp. pianists). 'Arthritic' finger pain, also seen in artists / sculptors.

Referred pain patterns
First dorsal interossei: strong finger pain in dorsum of index finger (lateral half), with vague pain on palmar surface and dorsum of hand. Other dorsal interossei: referred pain to the specific associated finger.
Lumbricales: pattern is similar to interossei.
Abductor digiti minimi: pain in dorsum of little finger.

Differential diagnosis
Cervical radiculopathy. Ulnar neuritis. Thoracic outlet syndrome. Digital nerve entrapment. Articular dysfunction.

Also consider
Intrinsic thumb muscles. Scalenes. Latissimus dorsi. Long finger flexors and / or extensors. Pectoralis major. Lateral and / or medial head of triceps brachii.

Advice to patient
Stretching and exercising. Examine work postures / ergonomics. Explore sporting activities (e.g. grip in golf). Use of ergonomic pens / cutlery.

Techniques

Spray and stretch	✓	
Injections	✓	✓

Dry needling	✓	
Trigger point release	✓	

9
Muscles of the Hip and Thigh

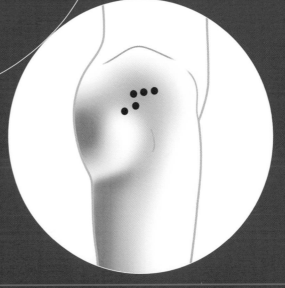

GLUTEUS MAXIMUS

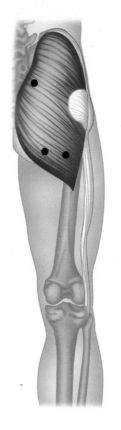

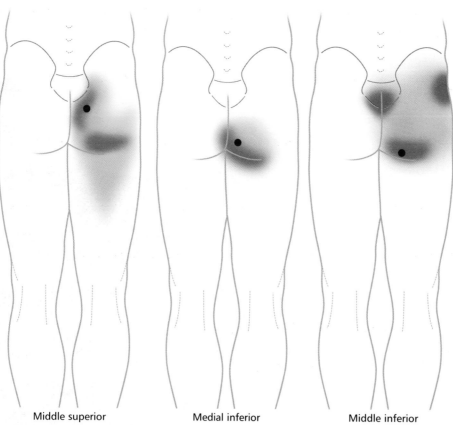

Middle superior   Medial inferior   Middle inferior

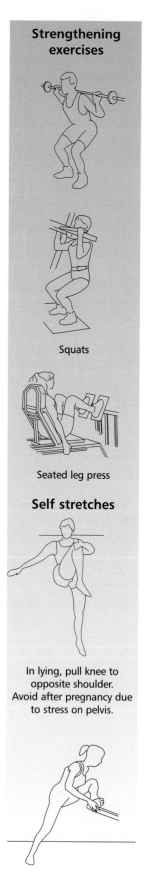

Strengthening exercises

Squats

Seated leg press

Self stretches

In lying, pull knee to opposite shoulder. Avoid after pregnancy due to stress on pelvis.

Greek, *gloutos*, buttock; *maximus*, biggest.

The gluteus maximus is the most coarsely fibred and heaviest muscle in the body, forming the bulk of the buttock.

Origin
Outer surface of ilium behind posterior gluteal line and portion of bone superior and posterior to it. Adjacent posterior surface of sacrum and coccyx. Sacrotuberous ligament. Aponeurosis of erector spinae.

Insertion
Deep fibres of distal portion: gluteal tuberosity of femur.
Remaining fibres: iliotibial tract of fascia lata.

Action
Upper fibres: laterally rotate hip joint. May assist in abduction of hip joint.
Lower fibres: extend and laterally rotate hip joint (forceful extension as in running or rising from sitting). Extend trunk. Assists in adduction of hip joint.
Through its insertion into the iliotibial tract, helps to stabilize the knee in extension.

Nerve
Inferior gluteal nerve, L5, S1, **2**.

Basic functional movement
Examples: Walking upstairs. Rising from sitting.

Indications
Pain on sitting. Pain walking (up hill). Pain on flexion. Buttock pain when swimming. Buttock pain after a fall or trip. Night pain. Restricted hip / thigh flexion. Listing gait. Cramping in cold.

Referred pain patterns
Three to four strong zones of pain in the buttock, with intercommunicating diffuse pain, occasionally just below (5–8cm) gluteal fold.

Differential diagnosis
Coccydynia. Pelvic inflammatory disease. Lower lumbar discopathy. Sacroiliitis. Bursitis (ischial tuberosity / trochanteric). Mechanical low back pain.

Also consider
Other gluteal muscles. Quadratus lumborum. Pubococcygeus. Hamstring muscles (attachment trigger points).

Advice to patient
Warmth and stretching. Gait and posture analysis. Pillow between knees when sleeping. Stretching programme. Swimming (not crawl).

Techniques

Spray and stretch	✓ ✓	Dry needling ✓ ✓
Injections	✓ ✓	Trigger point release ✓ ✓

TENSOR FASCIAE LATAE

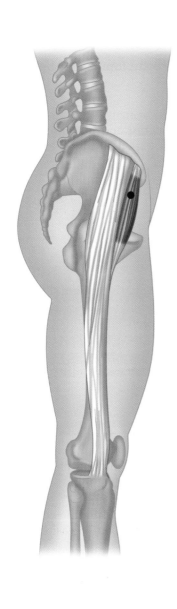

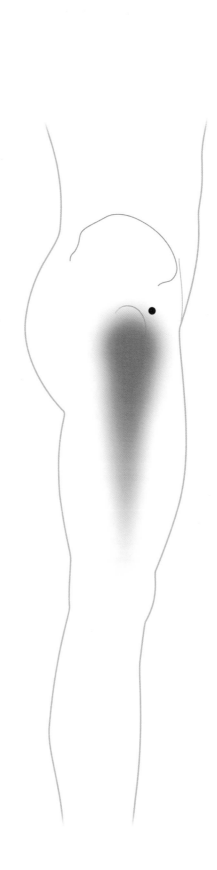

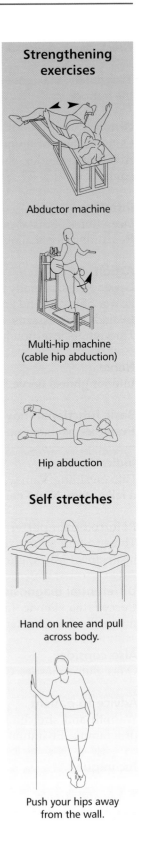

Strengthening exercises

Abductor machine

Multi-hip machine
(cable hip abduction)

Hip abduction

Self stretches

Hand on knee and pull
across body.

Push your hips away
from the wall.

Latin, *tensor*, stretcher, puller; *fascia(e)*, band(s); *latae*, broad.

This muscle lies anterior to gluteus maximus, on the lateral side of the hip.

Origin
Anterior part of outer lip of iliac crest, and outer surface of anterior superior iliac spine.

Insertion
Joins iliotibial tract just below level of greater trochanter.

Action
Flexes, abducts and medially rotates the hip joint. Tenses the fascia lata, thus stabilizing the knee. Redirects the rotational forces produced by gluteus maximus.

Nerve
Superior gluteal nerve, L**4**, **5**, S**1**.

Basic functional movement
Example: Walking.

Indications
Hip and knee pain (lateral). Pain on side lying. Pain on fast walking. Hip replacement rehabilitation. Fracture of neck of femur rehabilitation.

Referred pain patterns
Strong elliptical zone of pain from greater trochanter inferolaterally towards fibula.

Differential diagnosis
Trochanteric bursitis. Osteoarthritic hip. Sacroiliitis. Lumbar spondylosis.

Also consider
Gluteus medius. Gluteus minimus. Vastus lateralis. Rectus femoris. Sartorius. Quadratus lumborum.

Advice to patient
Avoiding prolonged positions (flexion). Avoid habitual postures (cross-legged, or standing on one leg). Pillow between knees at night. Running style, gait, and posture assessment. Warm up. Stretch regularly.

Techniques

Spray and stretch	✓	✓	Dry needling	✓	✓
Injections	✓		Trigger point release	✓	✓

GLUTEUS MEDIUS

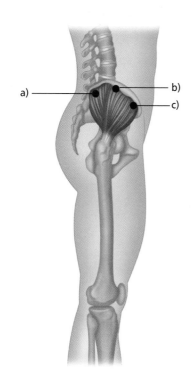

a)
b)
c)

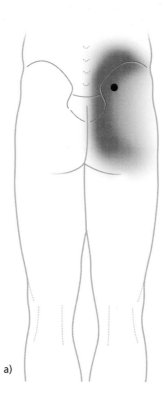

a)

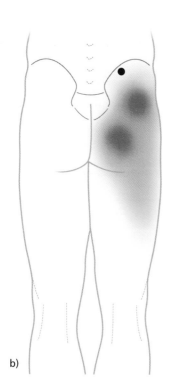

b)

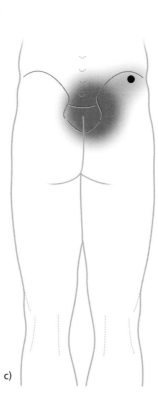

c)

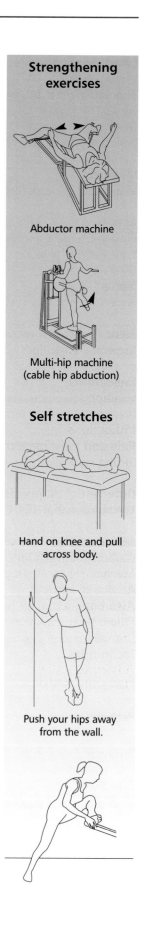

Strengthening exercises

Abductor machine

Multi-hip machine
(cable hip abduction)

Self stretches

Hand on knee and pull
across body.

Push your hips away
from the wall.

Greek, *gloutos*, buttock; *medius*, middle.

This muscle is mostly deep to and therefore obscured by gluteus maximus, but appears on the surface between gluteus maximus and tensor fasciae latae. During walking, this muscle, with gluteus minimus, prevents the pelvis from dropping towards the non weight-bearing leg.

Origin
Outer surface of ilium inferior to iliac crest, between the posterior gluteal line and the anterior gluteal line.

Insertion
Oblique ridge on lateral surface of greater trochanter of femur.

Action
Abducts the hip joint. Anterior fibres medially rotate and may assist in flexion of the hip joint. Posterior fibres slightly laterally rotate the hip joint.

Nerve
Superior gluteal nerve, L**4**, **5**, S**1**.

Basic functional movement
Example: Stepping sideways over an object such as a low fence.

Indications
Pain and tenderness in low back and buttocks. Night pain. Pain side lying. Post hip or spinal surgery. Sitting on wallet.

Referred pain patterns
Low back, medial buttock, sacral, and lateral hip radiating somewhat into the upper thigh.

Differential diagnosis
Radiculopathy (lumbosacral). Sacroiliitis. Hip joint dysfunction. Coccydynia. Greater tuberosity bursitis. Mechanical low back pain. Intermittent claudication.

Also consider
Quadratus lumborum. Other gluteal muscles. Pubococcygeus. Tensor fasciae latae. IT band. Piriformis. Lumbar erector spinae.

Advice to patient
Gait and posture analysis. Pillow between knees. Habitual postures. Stretching techniques.

Techniques

Spray and stretch	✓ ✓	Dry needling	✓	
Injections	✓ ✓	Trigger point release	✓ ✓	

GLUTEUS MINIMUS

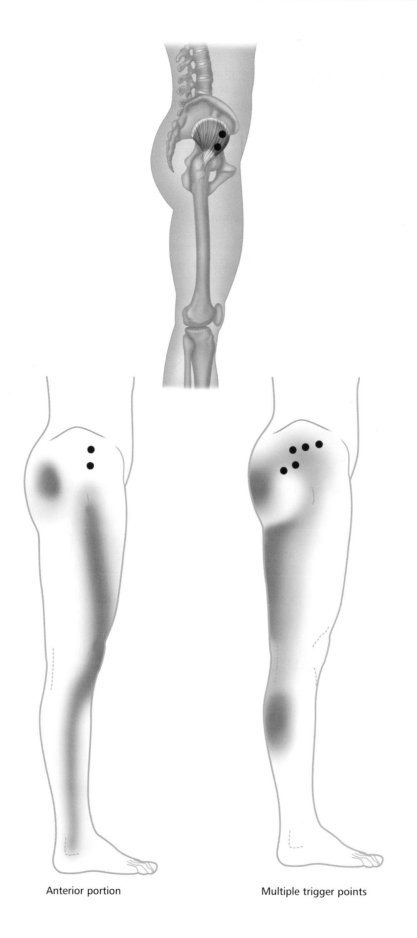

Anterior portion

Multiple trigger points

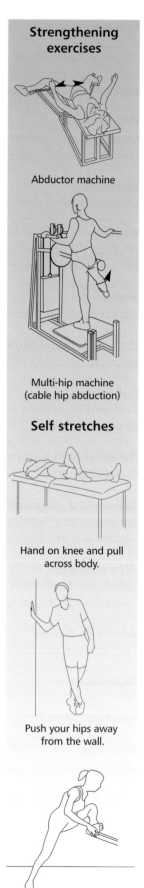

Strengthening exercises

Abductor machine

Multi-hip machine
(cable hip abduction)

Self stretches

Hand on knee and pull
across body.

Push your hips away
from the wall.

Greek, *gloutos*, buttock; *minimus*, smallest.

This muscle is situated anteroinferior and deep to gluteus medius, whose fibres obscure it.

Origin
Outer surface of ilium between anterior and inferior gluteal lines.

Insertion
Anterior border of greater trochanter.

Action
Abducts, medially rotates, and may assist in flexion of the hip joint.

Nerve
Superior gluteal nerve, L**4**, **5**, S**1**.

Basic functional movement
Example: Stepping sideways over an object such as a low fence.

Indications
Pain sitting to standing. Pain on walking. Pain at rest. Night pain (may wake). Pain on side lying. Hip replacement.

Referred pain patterns
A multipennate muscle with multiple anterior, middle, and posterior trigger points referring strong pain in lower buttock, hip, and lateral lower extremity beyond knee to ankle and calf.

Differential diagnosis
Radiculopathy (lumbar). Sacroiliitis. Hip joint dysfunction. Sciatic irritation. Hip bursitis.

Also consider
Tensor fasciae latae. Other gluteal muscles. Vastus lateralis. IT band. Quadratus lumborum. Peroneal muscles. Piriformis. Pelvic alignment.

Advice to patient
Self stretch techniques. Gait and posture. Habitual postures. Overload. Allow legs to 'hang' off the bed.

Techniques

Spray and stretch	✓	✓	Dry needling	✓	✓
Injections	✓	✓	Trigger point release	✓	✓

PIRIFORMIS

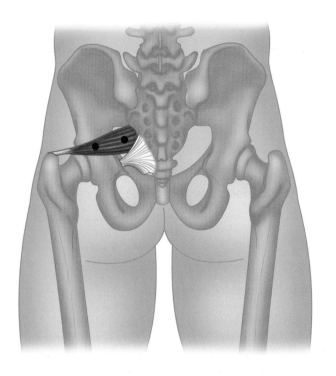

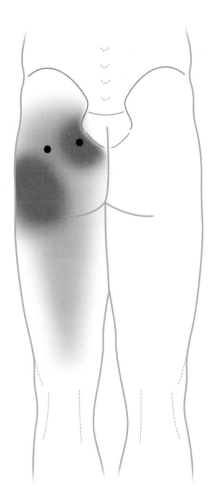

Strengthening exercise

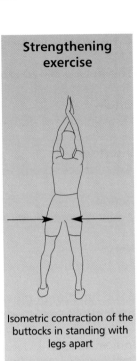

Isometric contraction of the buttocks in standing with legs apart

Self stretches

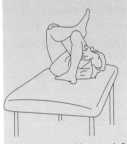

Cross right ankle over left knee and bring left knee slowly towards left shoulder, keeping the sacrum in contact with the ground or table. Be careful not to strain your knee joint.

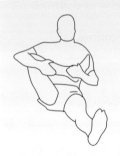

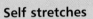

Latin, *pirum*, a pear, *piriform*, pear-shaped.

Piriformis leaves the pelvis by passing through the greater sciatic foramen.

Origin
Internal surface of sacrum. Sacrotuberous ligament.

Insertion
Superior border of greater trochanter of femur.

Action
Laterally rotates hip joint. Abducts the thigh when hip is flexed. Helps hold head of femur in acetabulum.

Nerve
Ventral rami of lumbar nerve, L(5) and sacral nerves, S**1**, **2**.

Basic functional movement
Example: Taking first leg out of car.

Indications
Constant 'deep' ache in buttock. Sciatica (pseudosciatica). Vascular compression posterior legs. Low back / buttock pain – worse for sitting. Often starts after a fall, or sitting on wallet with driving. Foot pain. Rectal pain. Sexual dysfunction (dyspareunia).

Referred pain patterns
Two strong zones of pain: 1) 3–4cm zone lateral to coccyx; 2) 7–10cm zone posterolateral buttock / hip joint +/- broad spill-over of diffuse pain between 1) and 2) and down thigh to above knee.

Differential diagnosis
Sacroiliitis. Lumbar radiculopathy. Coccydynia. Osteoarthritic hip. HLA (human leukocyte antigen) – B27 condition. Spinal stenosis. Discopathy (lumbar).

Also consider
Leg length discrepancy. Gluteal muscles. Quadratus lumborum. Attachment trigger point (origin) hamstrings. Gemelli. Obturators. Quadratus femoris. Levator ani. Coccygeus.

Advice to patient
Avoid habitual postures of cross-legged. Gait and posture analysis with reference to foot position. Driving position (foot). Self stretch. Use of self massage tools.

Techniques

Spray and stretch	✓		Dry needling	✓
Injections	✓	✓	Trigger point release	✓ ✓

HAMSTRINGS

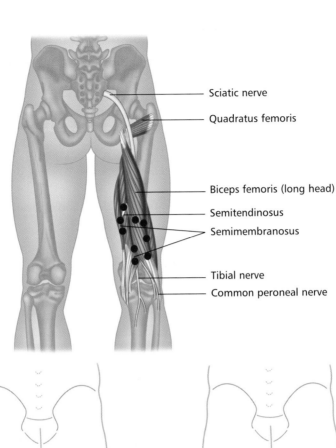

Sciatic nerve

Quadratus femoris

Biceps femoris (long head)

Semitendinosus

Semimembranosus

Tibial nerve

Common peroneal nerve

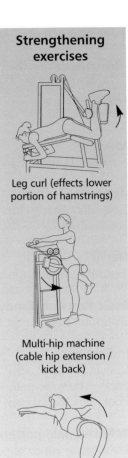

Strengthening exercises

Leg curl (effects lower portion of hamstrings)

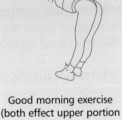

Multi-hip machine (cable hip extension / kick back)

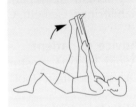

Good morning exercise (both effect upper portion of hamstrings)

Self stretches

Actively straighten your leg. For tighter hamstrings, hold onto a towel or strap slung over the sole of the foot.

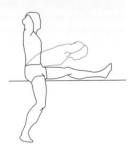

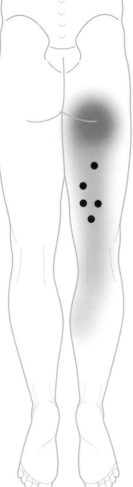

Semimembranosus / Semitendinosus

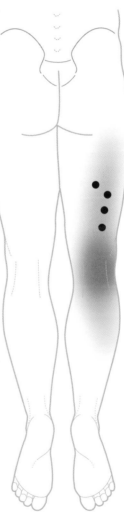

(short and long heads) Biceps femoris

German, *hamme*, back of leg; **Latin**, *stringere*, draw together.

The hamstrings consist of three muscles. From medial to lateral they are: semimembranosus, semitendinosus, and biceps femoris.

Origin
Ischial tuberosity (sitting bone). Biceps femoris also originates from the back of the femur.

Insertion
Semimembranosus: back of medial condyle of tibia (upper side part of tibia).
Semitendinosus: upper medial surface of shaft of tibia.
Biceps femoris: lateral side of head of fibula. Lateral condyle of tibia.

Action
Flex the knee joint. Extend the hip joint.
Semimembranosus and semitendinosus also medially rotate (turn in) the lower leg when knee is flexed.
Biceps femoris laterally rotates (turns out) the lower leg when the knee is flexed.

Nerve
Branches of the sciatic nerve, L4, **5**, S**1**, **2**, 3.

Basic functional movement
During running, the hamstrings slow down the leg at the end of its forward swing and prevent the trunk from flexing at the hip joint.

Indications
Posterior thigh pain in sitting and for walking (worse at night). Tenderness in back of legs may cause limping.

Referred pain patterns
Semimembranosus and semitendinosus: strong 10cm zone of pain, inferior gluteal fold, with diffuse pain posteromedial legs to Achilles tendon area.
Biceps femoris: diffuse pain, posteromedial legs with strong 10cm zone posterior to knee joint.

Differential diagnosis
Sciatica. Radiculopathy. Muscle tears. Osteitis. Bursitic osteoarthritis of knee. Knee joint dysfunction. Tenosynovitis.

Also consider
Piriformis. Popliteus. Gluteal muscles. Obturator internus. Vastus lateralis. Plantaris. Gastrocnemius.

Advice to patient
Regular stretching with hot and / or cold. Warm up and warm down before and after exercise. Hot showers / baths. Car seat posture. Work posture. Cycling positions.

Techniques

Spray and stretch	✓	✓	Dry needling	✓	✓
Injections	✓	✓	Trigger point release	✓	✓

ADDUCTORS

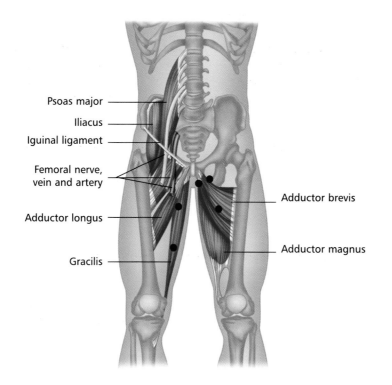

Psoas major

Iliacus

Iguinal ligament

Femoral nerve, vein and artery

Adductor longus

Gracilis

Adductor brevis

Adductor magnus

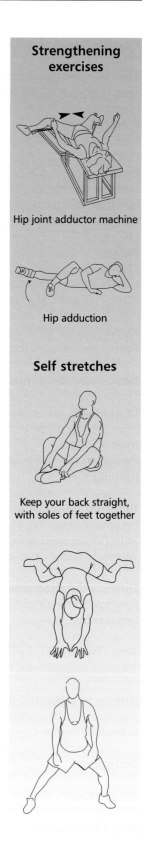
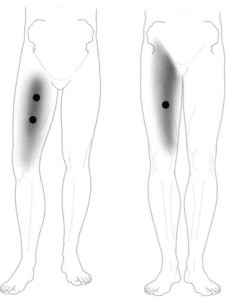

Adductor magnus

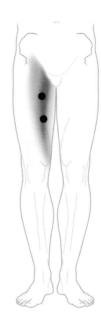

Adductor longus and brevis

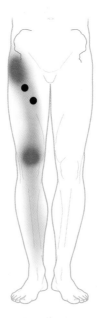

Gracilis

Latin, *adductor*, toward; *magnus*, large; *brevis*, short; *longus*, long.

The adductor magnus is the largest of the adductor muscle group, which also includes adductor brevis and adductor longus. Adductor longus is the most anterior of the three. Adductor brevis lies anterior to adductor magnus. The lateral border of the upper fibres of adductor longus form the medial border of the *femoral triangle* (sartorius forms the lateral boundary; the inguinal ligament forms the superior boundary).

Origin
Anterior part of pubic bone (ramus). Adductor magnus also takes origin from the ischial tuberosity.

Insertion
Whole length of medial side of femur, from hip to knee.

Action
Adduct and laterally rotate hip joint.
Adductors longus and brevis also flex the extended femur and extend the flexed femur.

Nerve
Magnus: posterior division of obturator nerve, L2, **3**, **4**. Tibial portion of sciatic nerve, L4, 5, S1.
Brevis: anterior division of obturator nerve, (L2–L4). Sometimes the posterior division also supplies a branch to it.
Longus: anterior division of obturator nerve, L**2**, **3**, 4.

Basic functional movement
Example: Bringing second leg in or out of car.

Indications
Deep pain and tenderness in medial thigh. Hip / leg stiffness on abduction. Pain on weight-bearing and / or rotating hip. 'Clicky' hip. Hot / stinging pain under thigh. Groin strain. Post hip replacement or fracture rehabilitation. Renal tubular acidosis. Legs swelling.

Referred pain patterns
There are several zones of referred pain: a) 2 zones localized around anterior hip 5–8cm, and above knee 5–8cm; b) whole anteromedial thigh from inguinal ligament to medial knee joint; c) medial thigh from hip to knee.

Differential diagnosis
Avulsion. Pubic symphysis dysfunction. Neuropathy. Lymphadenopathy. Hernia. Knee pain (mechanical). Osteoarthritic hip. Femoral herniation.

Also consider
Pectineus. Vastus medialis. Iliopsoas. Vastus lateralis. Sartorius (lower end).

Advice to patient
Home stretch programme. Avoid overuse at gym. Explore habitual postures. Skiing / cycling techniques. Vitamin / mineral deficiency.

Techniques

Spray and stretch	✓ ✓	Dry needling ✓ ✓
Injections	✓ ✓	Trigger point release ✓ ✓

PECTINEUS

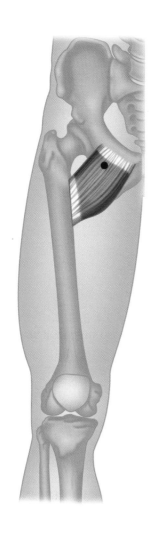

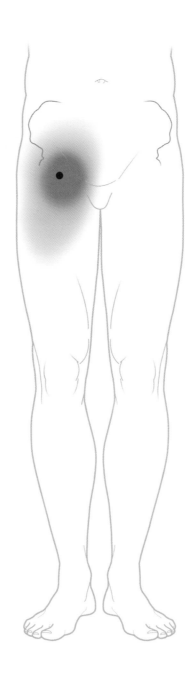

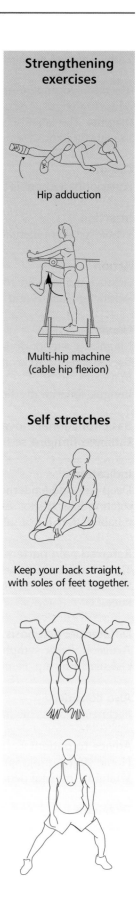

Strengthening exercises

Hip adduction

Multi-hip machine
(cable hip flexion)

Self stretches

Keep your back straight,
with soles of feet together.

Latin, *pecten*, comb, *pectenate*, shaped like a comb.

Pectineus is sandwiched between the psoas major and adductor longus.

Origin
Pecten of pubis, between iliopubic (iliopectineal) eminence and pubic tubercle.

Insertion
Pectineal line, from lesser trochanter to linea aspera of femur.

Action
Adducts the hip joint. Flexes the hip joint.

Nerve
Femoral nerve, L**2**, **3**, 4. Occasionally receives an additional branch from the obturator nerve, L3.

Basic functional movement
Example: Walking along a straight line.

Indications
Persistent 'internal' groin pain. Groin strain. Hip pain. Post hip replacement rehabilitation. Post hip fracture. Pregnancy. Postpartum. Pain during sexual intercourse. Pain during hip adduction exercises (gym).

Referred pain patterns
Strong 8–12cm zone of pain in anterior groin with more diffuse radiations in an oval – towards the anteromedial thigh.

Differential diagnosis
Inguinal hernia. Femoral hernia. Lymphadenopathy. Meralgia paresthetica. Lumbar radiculopathy. Vascular.

Also consider
Adductor longus and brevis. Iliopsoas. Limb length discrepancy.

Advice to patient
Avoid repetitive hip adduction and flexion, such as yoga positions (lotus). Avoid sitting cross-legged.

Techniques

Spray and stretch	✓		Dry needling		
Injections	✓	✓	Trigger point release	✓	✓

SARTORIUS

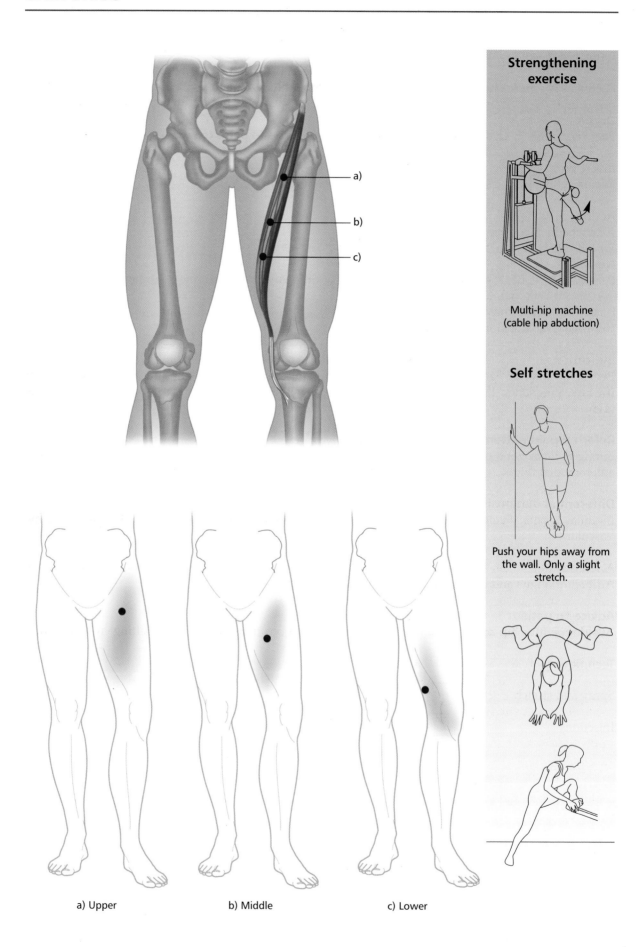

a)
b)
c)

Strengthening exercise

Multi-hip machine (cable hip abduction)

Self stretches

Push your hips away from the wall. Only a slight stretch.

a) Upper

b) Middle

c) Lower

Latin, tailor.

Sartorius is the most superficial muscle of the anterior thigh. It is also the longest strap muscle in the body. The medial border of the upper third of this muscle forms the lateral boundary of the femoral triangle (adductor longus forms the medial boundary; the inguinal ligament forms the superior boundary). The action of sartorius is to put the lower limbs in the cross-legged seated position of the tailor (hence its name from the Latin).

Origin
Anterior superior iliac spine and area immediately below it.

Insertion
Upper part of medial surface of tibia, near anterior border.

Action
Flexes hip joint (helping to bring leg forward in walking or running). Laterally rotates and abducts the hip joint. Flexes knee joint. Assists in medial rotation of the tibia on the femur after flexion. These actions may be summarized by saying that it places the heel on the knee of the opposite limb.

Nerve
Two branches from the femoral nerve, L**2**, **3**, (**4**).

Basic functional movement
Example: Sitting cross-legged.

Indications
Ache in anterior thigh. Sharp and / or tingling pain from hip to medial knee.

Referred pain patterns
Vague tingling from ASIS anteromedial medially across thigh towards medial knee joint.

Differential diagnosis
Meralgia parasthetica. Knee joint pathology. Lumbar radiculopathy. Inguinal lymphadenopathy. Vascular pathology. Inguinal and / or femoral hernia.

Also consider
Vastus medialis. Biceps femoris. Gracilis. Pectineus. Tensor fasciae latae.

Advice to patient
Gait and posture analysis. Prolonged sitting positions with knees crossed. Habitual postures. Can be overactive secondary to obesity and / or exercise (e.g. running with foot everted). Stretching exercises. Pillow between knees.

Techniques

Spray and stretch	✓	✓	Dry needling	✓	✓
Injections	✓	✓	Trigger point release	✓	✓

QUADRICEPS

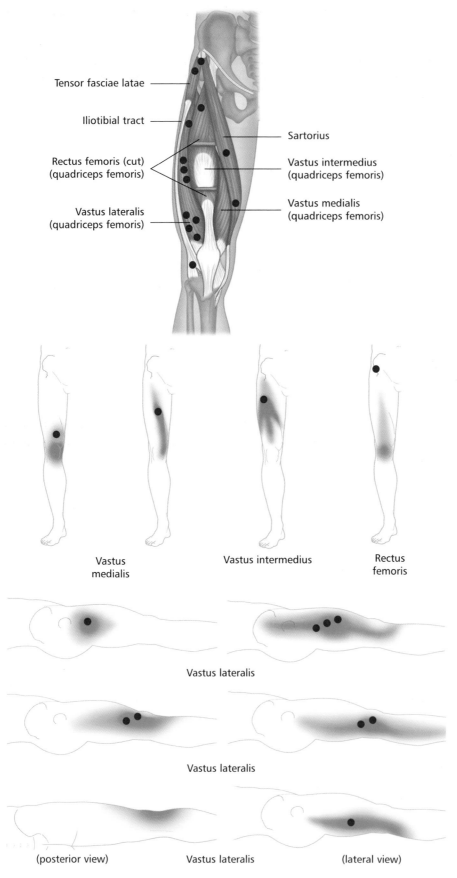

Tensor fasciae latae

Iliotibial tract

Sartorius

Rectus femoris (cut)
(quadriceps femoris)

Vastus intermedius
(quadriceps femoris)

Vastus lateralis
(quadriceps femoris)

Vastus medialis
(quadriceps femoris)

Vastus
medialis

Vastus intermedius

Rectus
femoris

Vastus lateralis

Vastus lateralis

(posterior view)   Vastus lateralis   (lateral view)

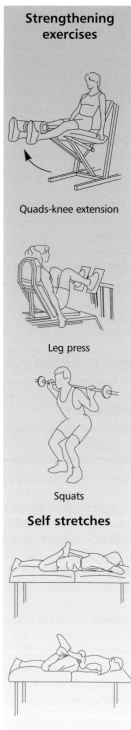

Strengthening exercises

Quads-knee extension

Leg press

Squats

Self stretches

Use opposite hand to hold
your ankle, or wrap a towel
around your leg and use
both hands.

Latin, *quadriceps*, four-headed; *rectum*, straight; *femoris*, of the thigh; *vastus*, great or vast; *lateral*, to the side; *medial*, middle; *intermedial*, between the middle.

The four quadriceps muscles are: rectus femoris, vastus lateralis, vastus medialis, and vastus intermedius. They all cross the knee joint, but the rectus femoris is the only one with two heads of origin and that also crosses the hip joint. The quadriceps straighten the knee when rising from sitting, during walking, and climbing. The vasti muscles as a group pay out to control the movement of sitting down.

Origin
Vastus group: upper half of shaft of femur.
Rectus femoris: front part of ilium (anterior inferior iliac spine). Area above hip socket.

Insertion
Patella, then via patellar ligament into the upper anterior part of the tibia (tibial tuberosity).

Action
Vastus group: extends the knee joint.
Rectus femoris: extends the knee joint, and flexes the hip joint (particularly in combination, as in kicking a ball).

Nerve
Femoral nerve, L**2**, **3**, **4**.

Basic functional movement
Examples: Walking up stairs. Cycling.

Indications
Pain and weakness in thigh. 'Giving way' of knee. Night pain. Pain on knee extension. Post hip fracture. Post femoral fracture and splinting. Decreased femoropatellar joint 'glide'. Pain on weight-bearing. Unexplained knee pain in young.

Referred pain patterns
Anterior, medial and / or lateral thigh pain. Vastus lateralis has many points of pain referral.

Differential diagnosis
IT band syndrome. Femoropatellar joint dysfunction. Quadriceps expansion injury. Tendonitis. Lumbar radiculopathy. Femoral nerve pathology. Knee problems / dysfunction (multipennate).

Also consider
Iliopsoas. Tensor fasciae latae. Gluteal muscle group. Sartorius.

Advice to patient
Correct lifting techniques. Tubigrip™. Avoid prolonged immobility. Home self stretch. Gait and posture assessment. Avoid heavy 'squats' in gym. Moist heat, cold or hot bath and stretch. Resting periods for cycling. Avoid habitual sitting (i.e. on feet, tucked under). Sleep with pillow between knees.

Techniques

| Spray and stretch | ✓ | ✓ | Dry needling | ✓ | ✓ |
| Injections | ✓ | ✓ | Trigger point release | ✓ | ✓ |

10

Muscles of the Leg and Foot

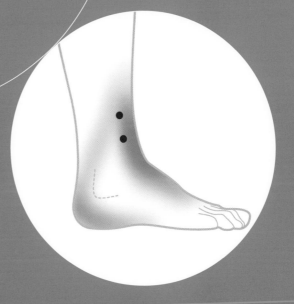

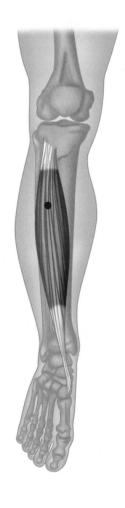

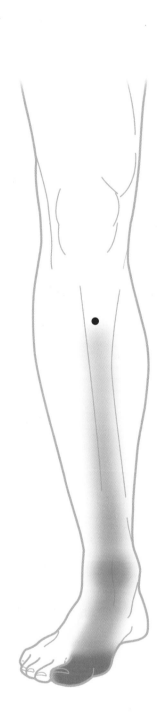

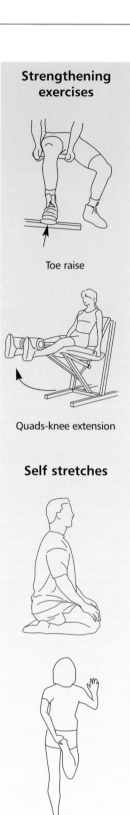

Strengthening exercises

Toe raise

Quads-knee extension

Self stretches

Latin, *tibia*, pipe or flute / shinbone; *anterior*, before.

Origin
Lateral condyle of tibia. Upper half of lateral surface of tibia. Interosseous membrane.

Insertion
Medial and plantar surface of medial cuneiform bone. Base of first metatarsal.

Action
Dorsiflexes the ankle joint. Inverts the foot.

Nerve
Deep peroneal nerve, L4, **5**, S1.

Basic functional movement
Example: Walking and running (helps prevent the foot from slapping onto the ground after the heel strikes. Lifts the foot clear of the ground as the leg swings forward).

Indications
Ankle pain and tenderness. Pain in the big toe. Shin splints (anterior tibial compartment syndrome). Foot dragging. Ankle weakness (children).

Referred pain patterns
Anteromedial vague pain along shin, with zone of pain 3–5cm in ankle joint (anterior) culminating in big toe pain (whole toe).

Differential diagnosis
Lumbar discopathy. Arthritic toes. Anterior tibial compartment syndrome. Shin splints (anterior). Varicose veins.

Also consider
Extensor hallucis longus. Peroneus tertius. Extensor hallucis brevis. Extensor digitorum brevis. Extensor digitorum longus. Flexor hallucis longus. First dorsal interosseous.

Advice to patient
Avoid prolonged car journeys and use of pedals. Change running surface and running shoes. Avoid walking (prolonged) on sloping surfaces. Have stretch programme (heat / warmth / cold). Adjust car seat. Use wedge under heel of foot for driving pedal.

Techniques

Spray and stretch	✓	✓	Dry needling	✓	✓	
Injections	✓	✓	Trigger point release	✓	✓	

EXTENSOR DIGITORUM LONGUS / EXTENSOR HALLUCIS LONGUS

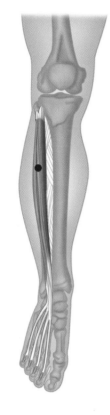

Extensor digitorum longus

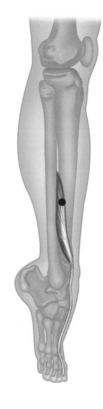

Extensor hallucis longus

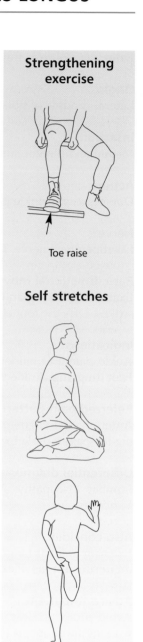

Strengthening exercise

Toe raise

Self stretches

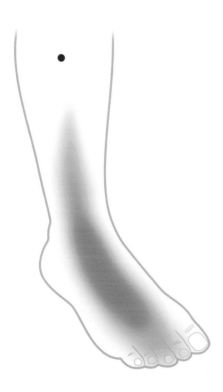

Extensor digitorum longus

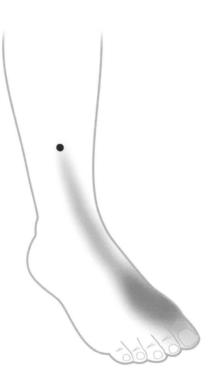

Extensor hallucis longus

Latin, *extensor*, to extend; *digit*, toe; *hallux*, big toe; *longus*, long.

Like the corresponding tendons in the hand, the extensor digitorum longus forms extensor hoods on the dorsum of the proximal phalanges of the foot. These hoods are joined by the tendons of the lumbricales and extensor digitorum brevis, but not by the interossei. The extensor hallucis longus lies between and deep to tibialis anterior and extensor digitorum longus.

Origin
Extensor digitorum longus: lateral condyle of tibia. Upper two-thirds of anterior surface of fibula. Upper part of interosseous membrane.
Extensor hallucis longus: middle half of anterior surface of fibula and adjacent interosseous membrane.

Insertion
Extensor digitorum longus: along dorsal surface of the four lateral toes. Each tendon dividing to attach to the bases of the middle and distal phalanges.
Extensor hallucis longus: base of distal phalanx of great toe.

Action
Extensor digitorum longus: extends toes at the metatarsophalangeal joints. Assists the extension of the interphalangeal joints. Assists in dorsiflexion of ankle joint and eversion of the foot.
Extensor hallucis longus: extends all the joints of the big toe. Dorsiflexes the ankle joint. Assists in inversion of the foot.

Nerve
Fibular (peroneal) nerve, L**4**, **5**, S**1**.

Basic functional movement
Example: Walking up the stairs (ensuring the toes clear the steps).

Indications
Dorsal foot pain. Metatarsalgia. Big toe pain (pain is 'persistent'). Night cramps.

Referred pain patterns
Extensor digitorum longus: pain in dorsum of foot extending to middle three toes.
Extensor hallucis longus: pain over big toe dorsum.

Differential diagnosis
Hammer toes. Claw toes. Bunions. Lesions of fibular head. Compartment syndromes. Foot drop (upper motor neurone). Tendonitis. Tendon damage.

Also consider
Peroneal muscles. Tibialis anterior.

Advice to patient
Footwear. Gait. Foot position during driving / sleeping. Orthotics. Review weight bearing exercises. Occupational postures.

Techniques

Spray and stretch	✓	✓	Dry needling	✓	✓
Injections	✓	✓	Trigger point release	✓	✓

FIBULARIS (PERONEUS) LONGUS, BREVIS, TERTIUS

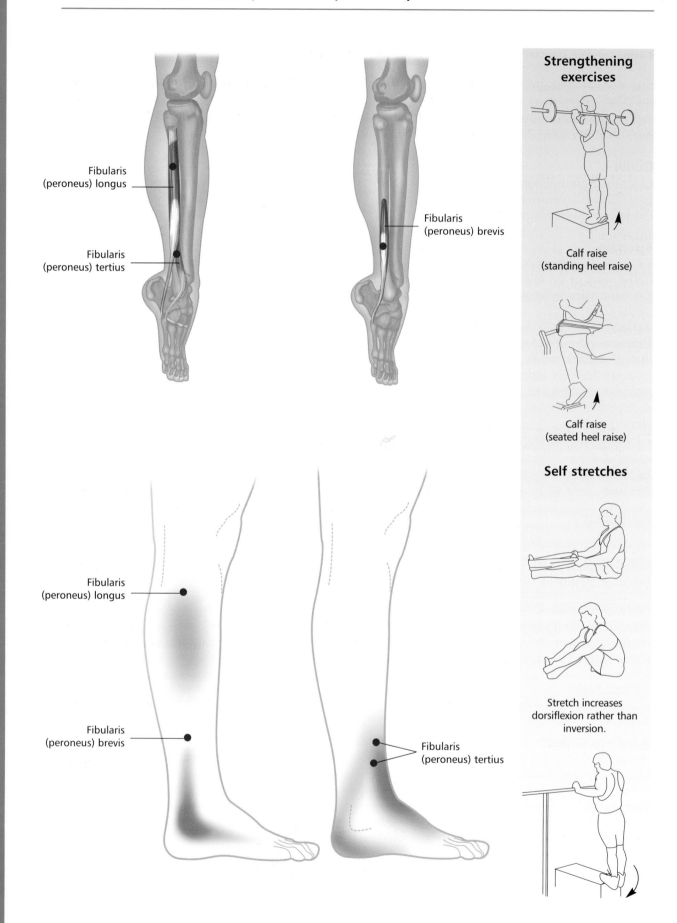

Fibularis (peroneus) longus

Fibularis (peroneus) tertius

Fibularis (peroneus) brevis

Fibularis (peroneus) longus

Fibularis (peroneus) brevis

Fibularis (peroneus) tertius

Strengthening exercises

Calf raise (standing heel raise)

Calf raise (seated heel raise)

Self stretches

Stretch increases dorsiflexion rather than inversion.

Latin, *fibula*, pin / buckle; *longus*, long; *brevis*, short; *tertius*, third.

The course of the tendon of insertion of fibularis longus helps maintain the transverse and lateral longitudinal arches of the foot. A slip of muscle from fibularis brevis often joins the long extensor tendon of the little toe, whereupon it is known as *peroneus digiti minimi*. Fibularis tertius is a partially separated lower lateral part of extensor digitorum longus.

Origin
Longus: upper two-thirds of lateral surface of fibula. Lateral condyle of tibia.
Brevis: lower two-thirds of lateral surface of fibula. Adjacent intermuscular septa.
Tertius: lower third of anterior surface of fibula and interosseous membrane.

Insertion
Longus: lateral side of medial cuneiform. Base of first metatarsal.
Brevis: lateral side of base of fifth metatarsal.
Tertius: dorsal surface of base of fifth metatarsal.

Action
Longus: everts foot. Assists plantar flexion of ankle joint.
Brevis: everts ankle joint.
Tertius: dorsiflexes ankle joint. Everts the foot.

Nerve
Fibular (peroneal) nerve, L**4**, **5**, S**1**.

Basic functional movement
Examples: Walking and running. Walking on uneven surfaces.

Indications
Pronation of feet. Repetitive inversion / eversion injury. Tenderness around malleolus. Ankle weakness. Post fracture (and casting) rehabilitation. Foot problems such as calluses, verrucas, neuromas. Osteoarthritis of the toes. Metatarsalgia.

Referred pain patterns
Mainly over lateral malleolus anteriorly and posteriorly in a linear distribution. Laterally along foot, occasionally vague pain in middle third of lateral aspect of lower leg.

Differential diagnosis
Rupture. Fracture of foot. Fracture of first metatarsal (styloid process). Foot problems. Fibular head dysfunction (common peroneal nerve). Toe problems. Ankle problems (arthritis). Gait dysfunction. Compartment syndromes (lateral). Osteoarthritis of hip.

Also consider
Tensor fasciae latae. Gluteus minimus. Extensor digitorum longus. Extensor hallucis brevis. Extensor digitorum brevis.

Advice to patient
Avoid high-heeled, and flat shoes. Regular stretching with hot and / or cold. Strapping / ankle support. Use of heel wedges and / or orthotics. Posture and gait advice. Examine shoes.

Techniques

Spray and stretch	✓	✓	Dry needling	✓	
Injections	✓	✓	Trigger point release	✓	✓

GASTROCNEMIUS

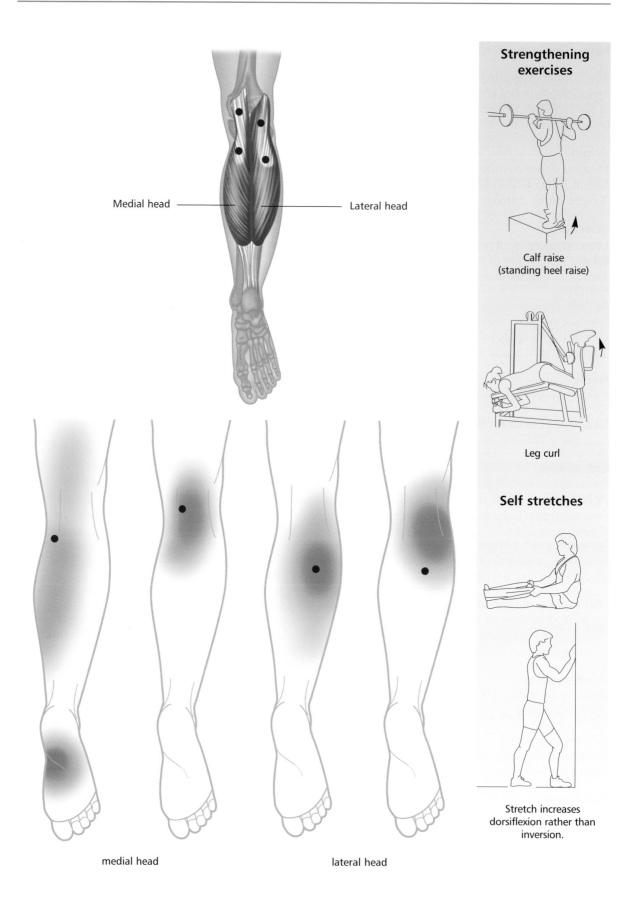

Medial head — — Lateral head

medial head

lateral head

Strengthening exercises

Calf raise
(standing heel raise)

Leg curl

Self stretches

Stretch increases
dorsiflexion rather than
inversion.

Greek, *gaster*, stomach; *kneme*, leg.

Gastrocnemius is part of the composite muscle known as *triceps surae*, which forms the prominent contour of the calf. The triceps surae comprises: gastrocnemius, soleus and plantaris. The popliteal fossa at the back of the knee is formed inferiorly by the bellies of gastrocnemius and plantaris, laterally by the tendon of biceps femoris, and medially by the tendons of semimembranosus and semitendinosus.

Origin
Medial head: popliteal surface of femur above medial condyle.
Lateral head: lateral condyle and posterior surface of femur.

Insertion
Posterior surface of calcaneus (via the tendo calcaneus; a fusion of the tendons of gastrocnemius and soleus).

Action
Plantar flexes foot at ankle joint. Assists in flexion of knee joint. It is a main propelling force in walking and running.

Nerve
Tibial nerve, S**1**, **2**.

Basic functional movement
Example: Standing on tip-toes.

Indications
Calf pain and stiffness. Nocturnal cramps. Foot pain (instep). Pain in back of knee on mechanical activity.

Referred pain patterns
Several trigger points in each muscle belly and attachment trigger point at ankle. The four most common points are indicated diagrammatically for medial and lateral heads.

Differential diagnosis
Thrombophlebitis. Deep vein thrombosis (varicose veins, intermittent claudication). S1 radiculopathy. Baker's cyst. Posterior tibial compartment syndrome. Achilles tendonitis. Sever's disease. Bursitis.

Also consider
Soleus. Plantaris. Tibialis posterior. Toe flexors (long). Toe extensors. Tibialis anterior.

Advice to patient
Avoid high-heeled shoes. Regular stretching. Warm up and warm down with exercise. Use cold and stretch / warmth and stretch. Change running shoes regularly. Posture.

Techniques

| Spray and stretch | ✓ | ✓ | Dry needling | ✓ | ✓ |
| Injections | ✓ | ✓ | Trigger point release | ✓ | ✓ |

PLANTARIS

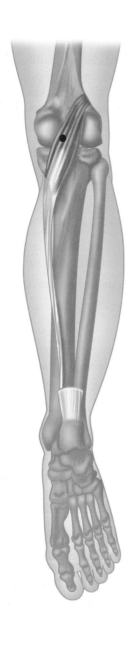

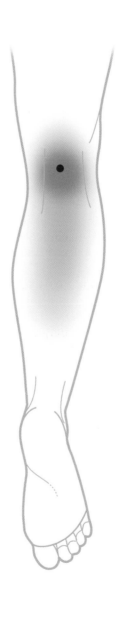

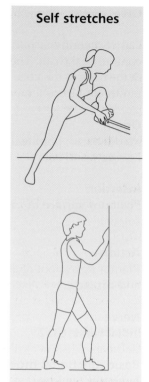

Self stretches

Stretch increases dorsiflexion rather than inversion.

Latin, *planta*, sole of the foot.

Part of the *triceps surae*. Its long slender tendon is equivalent to the tendon of palmaris longus in the arm.

Origin
Lower part of lateral supracondylar ridge of femur and adjacent part of its popliteal surface. Oblique popliteal ligament of knee joint.

Insertion
Posterior surface of calcaneus (or sometimes into the medial surface of the tendo calcaneus).

Action
Plantar flexes ankle joint. Feebly flexes knee joint.

Nerve
Tibial nerve, L4, **5**, **S1**, (2).

Basic functional movement
Example: Standing on tip-toes.

Indications
Calf pain. Heel pain. Posterior knee pain. Chronic and long-term use of high-heeled shoes.

Referred pain patterns
Popliteal fossa pain in 2–3cm zone radiating 5–10cm inferiorly into calf.

Differential diagnosis
Achilles tendonitis. Compartment syndrome. Vascular disease. Heel spur. Fasciitis. Subtalar joint problems. Venous pump mechanisms. Tendon rupture. Baker's cyst. Shin splints. Stress fracture. Leg length discrepancy.

Also consider
Popliteus. Gastrocnemius. Tibialis posterior. Quadratus plantae (of foot). Abductor hallucis (of foot).

Advice to patient
Change footwear. Change and vary running techniques and running surface. Change / avoid high heeled shoes. Regular stretching. Leg rests at home and at work. Use of cold. Massage after sports and warm up and warm down. Posture.

Techniques

Spray and stretch	✓	✓	Dry needling		
Injections	✓		Trigger point release	✓	✓

SOLEUS

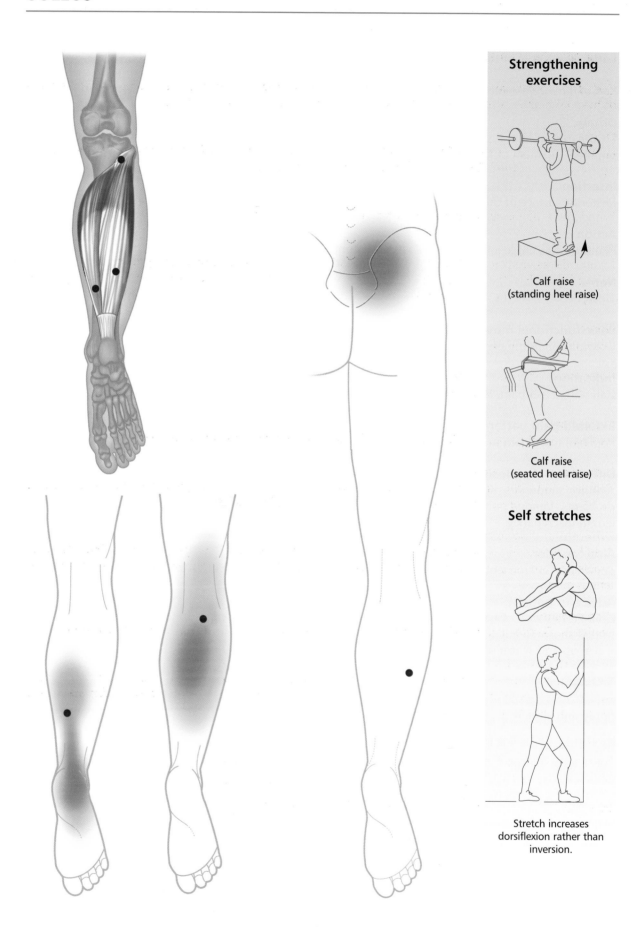

Strengthening exercises

Calf raise
(standing heel raise)

Calf raise
(seated heel raise)

Self stretches

Stretch increases
dorsiflexion rather than
inversion.

Latin, sole-shaped (fish).

Part of the *triceps surae*. The soleus is so called because its shape resembles a fish. The calcaneal tendon of the soleus and gastrocnemius is the thickest and strongest tendon in the body.

Origin
Posterior surfaces of head of fibula and upper third of body of fibula. Soleal line and middle third of medial border of tibia. Tendinous arch between tibia and fibula.

Insertion
With tendon of gastrocnemius into posterior surface of calcaneus.

Action
Plantar flexes ankle joint. The soleus is frequently in contraction during standing to prevent the body falling forwards at the ankle joint; i.e. to offset the line of pull through the body's centre of gravity. Thus, it helps to maintain the upright posture.

Nerve
Tibial nerve, L5, S**1**, **2**.

Basic functional movement
Example: Standing on tip-toes.

Indications
Calf pain. Heel pain. Posterior knee pain. Chronic and long-term use of high-heeled shoes.

Referred pain patterns
Pain in distal Achilles tendon and heel to the posterior half of foot. Calf pain from knee to just above Achilles tendon origin. 4–5cm zone of pain in sacroiliac region ipsilateral (rare).

Differential diagnosis
Achilles tendonitis. Compartment syndrome. Vascular disease. Heel spur. Fasciitis. Subtalar joint problems. Venous pump mechanisms. Tendon rupture. Baker's cyst. Shin splints. Stress fracture. Leg length discrepancy.

Also consider
Popliteus. Gastrocnemius. Tibialis posterior. Quadratus plantae (of foot). Abductor hallucis (of foot).

Advice to patient
Change footwear. Change and vary running techniques and running surface. Change / avoid high-heeled shoes. Regular stretching. Leg rests at home and at work. Use of cold. Massage after sports and warm up and warm down. Posture.

Techniques

| Spray and stretch | ✓ | ✓ | Dry needling | | |
| Injections | ✓ | | Trigger point release | ✓ | ✓ |

POPLITEUS

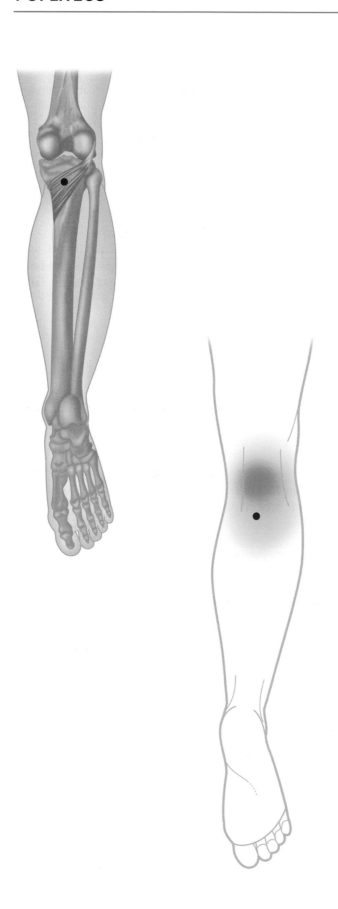

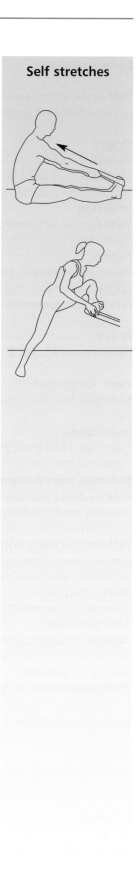

Self stretches

Latin, *poples*, ham.

The tendon from the origin of popliteus lies inside the capsule of the knee joint.

Origin
Lateral surface of lateral condyle of femur. Oblique popliteal ligament of knee joint.

Insertion
Upper part of posterior surface of tibia, superior to soleal line.

Action
Laterally rotates femur on tibia when foot is fixed on the ground. Medially rotates tibia on femur when the leg is non-weight bearing. Assists flexion of knee joint, (popliteus 'unlocks' the extended knee joint to initiate flexion of the leg). Helps reinforce posterior ligaments of knee joint.

Nerve
Tibial nerve, L**4**, **5**, S1.

Basic functional movement
Example: Walking.

Indications
Pain in back of knee in squatting, crouching, walking and / or running. Pain behind knee on walking uphill and going downstairs. Stiff knee on passive flexion and extension.

Referred pain patterns
Localized 5–6cm zone of pain (posterior and central knee joint) with some spreading of diffuse pain, radiating in all directions, especially inferiorly.

Differential diagnosis
Avulsion. Cruciate ligaments (instability). Baker's cyst. Osteoarthritis. Tendonitis. Cartilage (meniscus) injury. Vascular (deep vein thrombosis, thrombosis). Tenosynovitis.

Also consider
Hamstrings (biceps femoris). Gastrocnemius (ligamentum patellae). Plantaris.

Advice to patient
Avoid 'overload' on weight-bearing activities. Shoe orthotics. Stretching programme. Cycling position.

Techniques

Spray and stretch	✓ ✓	Dry needling	✓ ✓
Injections	✓	Trigger point release	✓

FLEXOR DIGITORUM LONGUS / FLEXOR HALLUCIS LONGUS

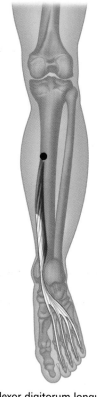

Flexor digitorum longus

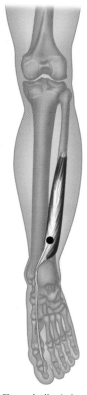

Flexor hallucis longus

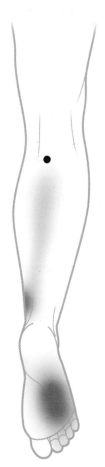

Flexor digitorum longus

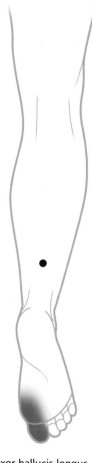

Flexor hallucis longus

Strengthening exercises

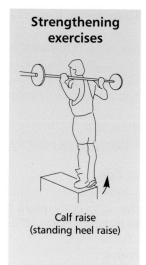

Calf raise
(standing heel raise)

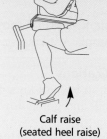

Calf raise
(seated heel raise)

Self stretches

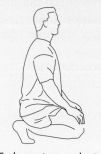

Curl your toes under to extend the toe joints.

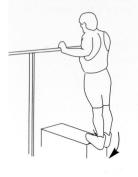

Keep your toes extended.

Latin, *flex*, to bend; *digit*, toe; *longus*, long; *hallux*, great toe.

The insertion of the tendons of flexor digitorum longus into the lateral four toes parallels the insertion of flexor digitorum profundus in the hand. Flexor hallucis longus helps maintain the medial longitudinal arch of the foot.

Origin
Flexor digitorum longus: medial part of posterior surface of tibia, below soleal line.
Flexor hallucis longus: lower two-thirds of posterior surface of fibula. Interosseous membrane. Adjacent intermuscular septum.

Insertion
Flexor digitorum longus: bases of distal phalanges of second through fifth toes.
Flexor hallucis longus: base of distal phalanx of great toe.

Action
Flexor digitorum longus: flexes all the joints of the lateral four toes. Helps to plantar flex the ankle joint and invert the foot.
Flexor hallucis longus: flexes all the joints of the great toe, and is important in the final propulsive thrust of the foot during walking. Helps to plantar flex the ankle joint and invert the foot.

Nerve
Tibial nerve, L5, S1, (2).

Basic functional movement
Walking / pushing off the surface in walking (esp. bare foot on uneven ground). Standing on tip-toes.

Indications
Foot pain on weight-bearing. Foot pain on uneven surfaces. Big toe pain.

Referred pain patterns
Flexor digitorum longus: vague linear pain in medial aspect of calf, with the main symptoms of plantar forefoot pain.
Flexor hallucis longus: strong pain in big toe, both plantar and into first metatarsal head.

Differential diagnosis
Shin splints. Compartment syndromes. Tendon ruptures. Instability of foot / ankle (medial). Stress (march) fracture. Morton's neuroma. Hammer toe / claw toe. Hallux valgus. Metatarsalgia. Osteoarthritis of first metatarsophalangeal joint. Gout. Plantar fasciitis.

Also consider
Superficial and deep intrinsic foot muscles. Tibialis posterior. Long and short extensors of toes.

Advice to patient
Examine / change in footwear. Gait and posture analysis. Regular stretching. Advice on running technique (e.g. run on flat surface).

Techniques

Spray and stretch	✓	✓	Dry needling	✓	
Injections	✓		Trigger point release	✓	✓

TIBIALIS POSTERIOR

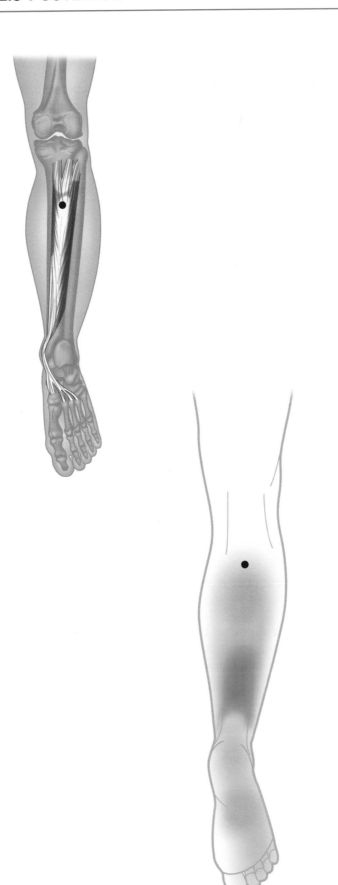

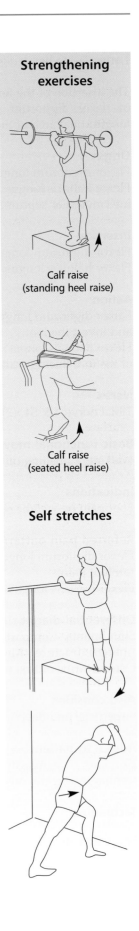

Strengthening exercises

Calf raise
(standing heel raise)

Calf raise
(seated heel raise)

Self stretches

Insertion

Abductor hallucis: medial side of base of proximal phalanx of great toe.

Flexor digitorum brevis: middle phalanges of second to fifth toes.

Abductor digiti minimi: lateral side of base of proximal phalanx of fifth toe.

Extensor digitorum brevis: base of proximal phalanx of great toe. Lateral sides of tendons of extensor digitorum longus to second, third and fourth toes.

Action

Abductor hallucis: abducts and helps flex great toe at metatarsophalangeal joint.

Flexor digitorum brevis: flexes all the joints of the lateral four toes except the distal interphalangeal joints.

Abductor digiti minimi: abducts fifth toe.

Extensor digitorum brevis: extends the joints of the medial four toes.

Nerve

Abductor hallucis, flexor digitorum brevis: medial plantar nerve, L4, **5**, S1.

Abductor digiti minimi: lateral plantar nerve, S**2**, 3.

Extensor digitorum brevis: deep fibular (peroneal) nerve, L4, **5**, S1.

Basic functional movement

Example: Facilitates walking. Helps foot stability and power in walking and running. Helping to gather up material under the foot by involving the big toe.

Indications

Foot pain (dorsal and plantar). 'Soreness' on walking, with 'aching' at rest. Pain on 'tip-toes'. Pain on weight-bearing, on 'initial' standing from sitting. Chronic high-heeled shoe wear.

Referred pain patterns

Abductor hallucis: medial heel pain radiating along the medial border of foot.

Flexor digitorum brevis: pain in plantar aspect of foot beneath (2–4th) metatarsal heads.

Abductor digiti minimi: pain in plantar aspect of foot beneath 5th metatarsal head.

Extensor digitorum brevis: have a strong oval overlapping zone of pain (4–5cm) in the lateral dorsum of foot just below the lateral malleolus.

Differential diagnosis

Avulsion fracture styloid process. Hallux valgus. Flat-footed. Hallux rigidus or hypermobility. Metatarsalgia. Hammer toe / claw toe deformity. Heel spur. Stress (march) fracture. Compartment syndromes. Varus and valgus of foot.

Also consider

Plantar interossei. Quadratus plantae. Adductor hallucis. Extensor digitorum longus. Extensor digitorum brevis. Flexor digitorum brevis. Hip, knee, ankle, and foot mechanics. Extensor hallucis brevis. Abductor hallucis.

Advice to patient

Gait and posture analysis. Footwear. Orthotics. Home stretching using a golf / tennis ball or rolling pin. Use a small heel. Warmth and stretch.

Techniques

| Spray and stretch | ✓ | ✓ | Dry needling | ✓ | |
| Injections | ✓ | ✓ | Trigger point release | ✓ | ✓ |

DEEP MUSCLES OF THE FOOT

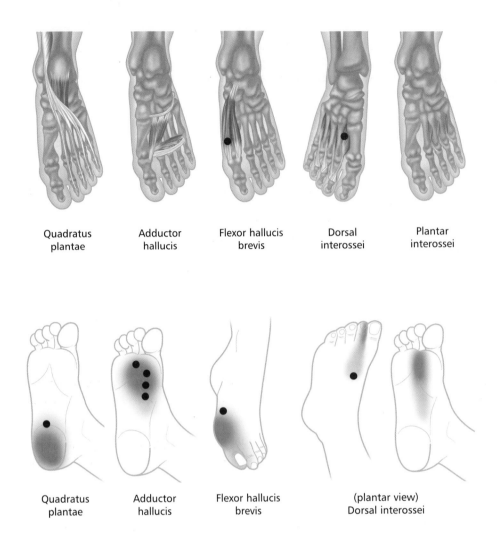

Quadratus
plantae

Adductor
hallucis

Flexor hallucis
brevis

Dorsal
interossei

Plantar
interossei

Quadratus
plantae

Adductor
hallucis

Flexor hallucis
brevis

(plantar view)
Dorsal interossei

Latin, *quadratus*, squared; *planta*, sole of the foot; *adduct*, toward; *hallux*, great toe; *flex*, to bend; *brevis*, short; *dorsum*, back; *interosseus*, between bones.

Comprising: quadratus plantae, adductor hallucis, flexor hallucis brevis, dorsal interossei, plantar interossei.

Origin
Quadratus plantae: medial head: medial surface of calcaneus; lateral head: lateral border of inferior surface of calcaneus.
Adductor hallucis: oblique head: bases of second, third and fourth metatarsals. Sheath of peroneus longus tendon; transverse head: plantar metatarsophalangeal ligaments of third, fourth and fifth toes. Transverse metatarsal ligaments.
Flexor hallucis brevis: medial part of plantar surface of cuboid bone. Adjacent part of lateral cuneiform bone. Tendon of tibialis posterior.
Dorsal interossei: adjacent sides of metatarsal bones.
Plantar interossei: bases and medial sides of third, fourth and fifth metatarsals.

Insertion
Quadratus plantae: lateral border of tendon of flexor digitorum longus.
Adductor hallucis: lateral side of base of proximal phalanx of great toe.
Flexor hallucis brevis: medial part: medial side of base of proximal phalanx of great toe; lateral part: lateral side of base of proximal phalanx of great toe.
Dorsal interossei: bases of proximal phalanges: first: medial side of proximal phalanx of second toe; second to fourth: lateral sides of proximal phalanges of second to fourth toes.
Plantar interossei: medial sides of bases of proximal phalanges of same toes.

Action
Quadratus plantae: flexes distal phalanges of second through to fifth toes. Modifies the oblique line of pull of the flexor digitorum longus tendons to bring it in line with the long axis of the foot.
Adductor hallucis: adducts and assists in flexing the metatarsophalangeal joint of the great toe.
Flexor hallucis brevis: flexes the metatarsophalangeal joint of the great toe.
Dorsal interossei: abduct (spread) toes. Flex metatarsophalangeal joints.
Plantar interossei: adduct (close together) toes. Flex metatatarsophalangeal joints.

Nerve
Quadratus plantae, adductor hallucis, dorsal interossei, plantar interossei: lateral plantar nerve, S**1**, **2**.
Flexor hallucis brevis: medial plantar nerve, L4, **5,** S1.

Basic functional movement
Example: Holding a pencil between the toes and the ball of the foot. Helping to gather up material under the foot by involving the big toe. Making a space between the big toe and the adjacent toe. Facilitates walking.

Indications
Foot pain. Heel pain. Pain in first metatarsophalangeal joint. Bunions / hallux valgus. Pain in second toe. Forefoot pain. Stiffness in tissues (inability to use orthotic support). Problems with walking. Numbness in foot. Hip / knee / ankle pain.

Referred pain patterns
Quadratus plantae: heel pain; adductor hallucis: forefoot pain; flexor hallucis brevis: pain around first metatarsophalangeal joint; dorsal / plantar interossei: second digit pain (antero-posterior).

Differential diagnosis
Morton's neuroma. Metatarsalgia. Plantar fasciitis. Heel spur. Stress fracture. Articular (joint) dysfunctions. Injured sesamoid bones. Lumbar radiculopathy (foot drop). Hallux valgus. Calcaneal compartment syndrome. Gout. Arthritis.

Also consider
Hip, knee, and ankle problems. Flexor digitorum brevis.

Advice to patient
Stretching with cold (and / or hot). Examine footwear (is it too tight?). Treat any joint dysfunctions. Stretching exercises / home stretch over tennis / golf ball. Proper orthotics. Gait and posture analysis.

Techniques

Spray and stretch	✓ ✓	Dry needling	✓
Injections	✓ ✓	Trigger point release	✓ ✓

Glossary of Medical Terms

Achilles tendonitis	Inflammation of the Achilles tendon.
Adhesive capsulitis	Adhesive inflammation between the joint capsule and the peripheral articular cartilage of the shoulder. Causes pain, stiffness, and limitation of movement. Also called frozen shoulder.
Angina	Any spasmodic, choking, or suffocative pain, e.g. preceding a myocardial infarction (heart attack).
Ankylosing spondylitis	Form of degenerative joint disease that affects the spine. Systemic illness, producing pain and stiffness as a result of inflammation of the sacroiliac, intervertebral, and costovertebral joints.
Anterior tibial compartment syndrome	Rapid swelling, increased tension, and pain of the anterior tibial compartment of the leg. Usually a history of excessive exertion.
Aortic aneurysm	Sac formed by the dilation of the wall of the aorta, which is filled with fluid or clotted blood.
Apley's scratch test	Determines range of motion: internal rotation and adduction; internal rotation, extension, and adduction; abduction, flexion, and external rotation.
Arteritis	Inflammation of an artery.
Arthropathy	Any joint disease.
Articular dysfunction	Disturbance, impairment, or abnormality of a joint.
Avulsion fracture	Indirect fracture caused by compressive forces from direct trauma or excessive tensile forces.
Baker's cyst	Swelling behind the knee, caused by leakage of synovial fluid which has become enclosed in a sac of membrane.
Barrett's syndrome	Peptic ulcer of the lower oesophagus, sometimes containing functional mucous cells, instead of the normal squamous cell epithelium.
Bruxism	Involuntary spasmodic gnashing, grinding, and clenching of teeth. Related to repressed aggression, emotional tension, etc.
Bunion	Abnormal prominence of the inner aspect of the first metatarsal head, resulting in displacement of the great toe (hallux valgus).
Bursa	Fibrous sac membrane containing synovial fluid, typically found between tendons and bones. It acts to reduce friction during movement.
Bursitis	Inflammation of the bursa, e.g. subdeltoid bursa.
Calcific tendonitis	Inflammation and calcification of the subacromial or subdeltoid bursa. This results in pain, and limitation of movement of the shoulder.
Capsulitis	Inflammation of a capsule, e.g. joint.
Cardiac arrhythmia	Variation from the normal rhythm of the heartbeat.
Carpal tunnel syndrome	Compression of the median nerve as it passes through the carpal tunnel, leading to pain and tingling in the hand.
Claw toe	Toe deformity, particularly in patients with rheumatoid arthritis, consisting of dorsal subluxation of toes 2–5; painful condition during walking. The patient develops a shuffling gait.

Coccydynia	Pain in the coccyx and neighbouring region. Also known as coccygodynia.
Compartment syndrome	Condition in which increased intramuscular pressure impedes blood flow and function of tissues within that compartment.
Complex regional pain syndrome	Syndrome of vascular changes secondary to autonomic nervous system dysfunction (vaso nervorum / vaso vasorum).
Deep vein thrombosis (DVT)	The formation of a stationary blood clot in the wall of one or more of the deep veins of the lower leg.
De Quervain's tenosynovitis	Inflammatory narrowing tenosynovitis of the abductor pollicis longus and extensor pollicis brevis tendons.
Dermomyotome	Zone of undifferentiated embryological tissue – pre-cursor of skin cells and muscle cells.
Dermatomyositis	Chronic, progressive inflammatory disease of skeletal muscle, occurring in association with characteristic inflammatory skin changes.
Discogenic pain	Pain caused by derangement of an intervertebral disc.
Discopathy	Disease of an intervertebral cartilage (disc).
Diverticular disease	Disease of a sac occurring normally or created by herniation of the lining mucous membrane through a defect in the muscular coat of a tubular organ.
Dupuytren's contracture	Shortening, thickening, and fibrosis of the palmar fascia, producing a flexion deformity of a finger / toe.
Dysmenorrhoea	Difficult or painful menstruation.
Dyspareunia	Difficult or painful sexual intercourse.
Dyspnoea	Breathlessness or shortness of breath.
Epicondylitis	Inflammation and microrupturing of the soft tissues on the epicondyles of the distal humerus.
Erythema	Redness of the skin produced by congestion of the capillaries.
Fasciitis	Inflammation of the fascia surrounding portions of a muscle.
Fibromyalgia	Pain and stiffness in the muscles and joints that is either diffuse or has multiple trigger points.
Frozen shoulder syndrome	*see* adhesive capsulitis.
Golfer's elbow	Inflammation of the medial epicondyle of the humerus caused by activities (e.g. golf) that involve gripping and twisting, especially when there is a forceful grip.
Gout	Condition caused by a build-up of uric acid in the body and affects the joints, most commonly the big toe joint.
Hallux rigidus	Painful flexion deformity of the great toe, in which there is limitation of motion at the metatarsophalangeal joint.
Hallux valgus	Angulation of the great toe away from the midline of the body, or toward the other toes.
Hammer toe	Flexion deformity of the distal interphalangeal (DIP) joint of the toes.
Heberdan's node	Small hard nodule(s), formed at the distal interphalangeal articulations of the fingers. Associated with interphalangeal osteoarthritis.
Heel spur	Boney spur from the calcaneum.
Hemiplegia	Paralysis of one side of the body.
Hernia	Protrusion of abdominal viscera through a weakened portion of the abdominal wall.

Herpes zoster	Acute infectious, usually self-limited, disease believed to represent activation of latent human herpes virus 3 in those who have been made partially immune after a previous attack of chickenpox.
HLA	Human leukocyte antigen.
Horner's syndrome	Sinking in of the eyeball, ptosis of the upper eyelid, slight elevation of the lower lid, flushing of the affected side of the face, and constriction of the pupil.
Impingement syndrome	Chronic condition caused by a repetitive overhead activity that damages the glenoid labrum, long head of the biceps brachii, and subacromial bursa.
IT band syndrome	Pain / inflammation of the iliotibial band, a non-elastic collagen cord stretching from the pelvis to below the knee. There are various biomechanical causes.
Kyphosis	Abnormal condition of the thoracic spine, characterized by increased convexity when viewed from the side.
Lesion	Any pathological or traumatic discontinuity of tissue or loss of function of a part.
Lordosis	Excessive convex curve in the lumbar region of the spine.
Lymphadenopathy	Disease of the lymph nodes.
Malocclusion	Malposition of the maxillary and mandibular teeth, affecting movements of the jaw that are essential for mastication.
McBurney's point	Site one-third the distance between the anterior superior iliac spine (ASIS) and umbilicus that, with deep palpation, produces rebound tenderness, indicating appendicitis.
Meralgia paresthetica	Entrapment of the lateral femoral cutaneous nerve at the inguinal ligament, causing pain and numbness of the outer surface of the thigh in the region supplied by the nerve.
Metatarsalgia	Condition involving general discomfort around the metatarsal's heads.
Morton's neuralgia	Form of foot pain, metatarsalgia caused by compression of a branch of the plantar nerve by the metatarsal heads.
Morton's neuroma	Tumour growing from a nerve or made up largely of nerve cells and nerve fibres, resulting from Morton's neuralgia.
Neuritis	Inflammation of a nerve, with pain and tenderness.
Neurogenic	Forming nervous tissue, or originating in the nervous system.
Neuropathy	Functional disturbance or pathological change in the peripheral nervous system.
Odynophagia	Pain caused by swallowing.
Oedema	Accumulation of lymphatic fluid in the tissues, caused by failure of the lymphatic system to drain properly.
Osteitis	Inflammation of a bone, causing enlargement of the bone, tenderness, and a dull, aching pain.
Osteoarthritis	Noninflammatory degenerative joint disease, characterized by degeneration of the articular cartilage, hypertrophy of bone at the margins, and changes in the synovial membrane. Seen particularly in older persons.

Paget's disease	Rare disease where bone is replaced by fibrous tissue that then becomes hard and brittle, with much pain. Particularly affecting the skull, spine, and leg bones.
Painful arc syndrome	Pain located within a limited number of degrees in the range of motion.
Polymyalgia rheumatica	Syndrome characterized by proximal joint and muscle pain. Affecting the elderly.
Posterior tibial compartment syndrome	Pain in the posterior compartment of the lower leg, including soleus, gastrocnemius, tibialis posterior, flexor digitorum longus, and flexor hallucis longus. Site of pain varies depending on muscles affected.
Postpartum	After childbirth, or delivery.
Ptosis	Downward displacement.
Radiculopathy	Disease of the nerve roots.
Repetitive strain injury (RSI)	Refers to any overuse condition, such as strain, or tendonitis in any part of the body.
Rheumatoid arthritis	Autoimmune disease, in which the immune system attacks the body's own tissues. Causes inflammation of many parts of the body.
Sacroiliitis	Inflammation (arthritis) in the sacroiliac joint.
Scalene syndrome	Thoracic outlet syndrome caused by compression of nerves and vessels between a cervical rib and scalenus anterior.
Scapulocostal syndrome	Pain in the superior or posterior aspect of the shoulder girdle, as a result of long-standing alteration of the relationship of the scapula and the posterior thoracic wall.
Sciatica	Compression of a spinal nerve due to a herniated disc, a muscle-related or facet joint disease, or compression between the two parts of the piriformis.
Scleroderma	Chronic hardening and thickening of the skin, occurring in a localized or focal form as well as a systemic disease.
Scoliosis	Lateral rotational spinal curvature.
Seronegative spondyloarthropathy	A general term comprising a number of degenerative joint diseases having common features, e.g. synovitis of the peripheral joints.
Sever's disease	A traction-type injury, or osteochondrosis, of the calcaneal apophysis, seen in young adolescents.
Spondyloarthropathy	Disease of the joints of the spine.
Spondylolisthesis	Forward displacement of one vertebra over another.
Spondylolysis	Dissolution of a vertebra.
Spondylosis	Degenerative spinal changes due to osteoarthritis.
Stenosis	Abnormal narrowing of a duct or canal, e.g. spinal stenosis, a narrowing of the vertebral canal, caused by encroachment of the bone upon the space.
Stress (march) fracture	Hairline crack of a bone caused by excessive repetitive stress.
Tendinopathy	Disease of a tendon.
Tendonitis	Inflammation of a tendon. Also known as tendinitis.
Tennis elbow	Tendonitis of the muscles of the back of the forearm at their insertion and is caused by excessive hammering or sawing type movements, or a tense, awkward grip on a tennis racquet.
Tenosynovitis	Inflammation of a tendon sheath.
Thoracic outlet syndrome	Compression of the brachial plexus rather than the nerve roots, and so symptoms appear in the arm instead of the neck.
Thrombophlebitis	Inflammation of a vein, associated with thrombus formation.

Thrombus	Stationary blood clot along the wall of a blood vessel, frequently causing vascular obstruction.
Tic douloureux	*see* trigeminal neuralgia.
Tietze's syndrome	Swellings of one or more costal cartilages, especially the second rib. The anterior chest pain may mimic that of coronary artery disease.
TMJ (temporomandibular joint) syndrome	Complex of symptoms including tinnitus, dizziness, headache, and clicking of the TMJ. Causes suggested include mandibular overclosure, and stress.
Trigeminal neuralgia	Excruciating episodic pain in the area supplied by the trigeminal nerve, often precipitated by stimulation of well-defined trigger points.
Trismus	Motor disturbance of the trigeminal nerve, especially spasm of the masticatory muscles, with difficulty in opening the mouth.
Urethritis	Inflammation of the urethra.
Valsalva's manoeuvre	Forcible exhalation effort against a closed glottis, or occluded nostrils and a closed mouth.
Varicocele	Condition in males characterized by varicosity of the veins in the skin of the scrotum. Accompanied by a constant dull pain.
Vertebral artery syndrome	Vascular insufficiency involving compression of the vertebral artery in the cervical spine.
Vestibule	Space or cavity at the entrance to a canal.
Vestibulocochlear	Pertaining to the vestibule of the ear and the cochlea.
Visceral pain	Pain resulting from injury or disease to an organ in the thoracic or abdominal cavity.

Resources

1. Caillet, R.: 1991. *Shoulder Pain.* F. A. Davis.

2. Chaitow, L.: 1996. *The Acupuncture Treatment of Pain.* Inner Traditions.

3. Davies, C.: 2004. *The Trigger Point Therapy Workbook, 2nd edition.* New Harbinger.

4. deJong, R. N.: 1967. *The Neurological Examination, 2nd & 3rd editions.* Harper & Row, New York.

5. Ferner, H., & Staubesand, J.: 1984. *Sabotta Atlas of Human Anatomy (vol. 10).* Lippincott, Williams & Wilkins, Baltimore.

6. Fishbain, D. A., Goldberg, M., & Meagher, B. R., et al.: 1986. Male and female chronic pain patients categorized by DSM-III psychiatric diagnostic criteria. *Pain* **26**: 181–197.

7. Foerster. O., & Bumke, O.: 1936. *Handbuch der Neurologie (vol. V).* Publisher unknown, Breslau.

8. Friction, J. R., Kroening, R., & Haley, D., et al.: 1985. Myofascial pain syndrome of the head and neck: a review of clinical characteristics of 164 patients. *Oral Surg.* **60**: 615–623.

9. Fröhlich, D., & Fröhlich, R.: 1995. Das Piriformiss syndrom: eine haufige Differential diagnose des lumboglutaalen Schmerzez (Pirifomis syndrome: A frequent item in the differential diagnosis of lumbogluteal pain). *Manuelle Medizin* **33**: 7–10.

10. Gerwin, R. D.: 1995. A study of 96 subjects examined both for fibromyalgia and myofascial pain (abstract). J. *Musculoskeletal Pain* **3** (1): 121.

11. Haymaker, W., & Woodhall, B.: 1953. *Peripheral Nerve Injuries, 2nd edition.* W. B. Saunders Co., Philadelphia.

12. Hecker, H., et al.: 2001. *Color Atlas of Acupuncture.* Thieme.

13. Jarmey, C.: 2004. *The Atlas of Musculo-skeletal Anatomy.* Lotus Publishing / North Atlantic Books, Chichester / Berkeley.

14. Juhan, D.: 1987. *Job's Body.* Station Hill Press.

15. Kendall, F. P., & McCreary, E. K.: 1983. *Muscles, Testing & Function, 3rd edition.* Lippincott, Williams and Wilkins, Baltimore.

16. Kuchera, W., & Kuchera, L.: 1994. *Osteopathic Principles in Practice.* Greyden Press.

17. Melzack, Fox & Shilwell, 1997. Journal unknown.

18. Romanes, G. J. (editor): 1972. *Cunningham's Textbook of Anatomy, 11th edition.* Oxford University Press, London.

19. Schultz, R., & Feitis, R.: 1996. *The Endless Web – Fascial Anatomy & Physical Reality.* North Atlantic Books, Berkeley.

20. Shankland, W.: 1996. *TMJ: Its Many Faces, Diagnosis of TMJ & Related Disorders, 2nd edition.* AN and DEM Inc.

21. Skelly, M., & Helm. A.: 1999. *Alternative Treatments for Fibromyalgia & Chronic Fatigue Syndrome.* Hunter House Publishing.

22. Skootsky, S. A., Jaeger. B., & Oye, R. K.: 1989. Prevalence of myofascial in general internal medicine practice. *West J. Med.* **151** : 157–160.

23. Spaleholz, W.: (date unknown). *Hand Atlas of Human Anatomy (vols. II & III, 6th edition).* J. B. Lippincott, London.

24. Starlanyl, D.J., & Copeland, M.E.: 2000. *Myofascial Pain & Dysfunction, Fibromyalgia & Chronic Myofascial Pain, a Survival Manual.* New Harbinger.

25. Travell, J & Simons, D.: 1999. *Myofascial Pain & Dysfunction: The Trigger Point Manual (vol. 1)*. Lippincott, Williams & Wilkins, Baltimore.

26. Travell, J & Simons, D.: 1993. *Myofascial Pain & Dysfunction: The Trigger Point Manual (vol. 2)*. Lippincott, Williams & Wilkins, Baltimore.

27. Zohn, D., & Mennell, J.M.: 1988. *Musculo-skeletal Pain: Diagnosis & Physical Treatment, 2nd edition*. Lippincott, Williams & Wilkins, Baltimore.

Additional Resources

Alter, M. J.: 1998. *Sport Stretch: 311 Stretches for 41 Sports*. Human Kinetics, Champaign.

Anderson, D. M. (chief Lexicographer): 2003. *Dorland's Illustrated Medical Dictionary, 30th edition*. Saunders, an imprint of Elsevier, Philadelphia.

Clemente, C. M. (editor): 1985. *Gray's Anatomy of the Human Body, 30th edition*. Lea & Febiger, Philadelphia.

Cook, B. B., and Stewart, G. W.: 1996. *Strength Basics*. Human Kinetics, Champaign.

Jarmey, C.: 2003. *The Concise Book of Muscles*. Lotus Publishing / North Atlantic Books, Chichester / Berkeley.

McAtee, R. E., and Charland, C.: 1999. *Facilitated Stretching, 2nd edition*. Human Kinetics, Champaign.

Norris, C. M.: 1999. *The Complete Guide to Stretching*. A & C Black, London.

Yessis, M.: 1992. *Kinesiology of Exercise*. Masters Press, Lincolnwood.

Index

Index of Muscles